The Quality System Compendium

GMP Requirements
& Industry Practice

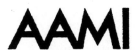

Association for the Advancement of Medical Instrumentation
1110 North Glebe Road, Suite 250, Arlington, VA 22201-5762
Phone 703-525-4890 / Fax 703-276-0793

Published by the
Association for the Advancement of Medical Instrumentation
1110 North Glebe Road, Suite 250
Arlington, VA 22201-5762

Printed in the United States of America

ISBN 1-57020-076-9

TABLE OF CONTENTS

ACCEPTANCE ACTIVITIES *(continued)*

MONITORING AND FEEDBACK/*page 135*

DOCUMENTS AND RECORDS/*page 155*

FOREWORD AND ACKNOWLEDGMENTS

The Quality System Compendium: GMP Requirements & Industry Practice is a comprehensive body of knowledge on the Food and Drug Administration's (FDA's) Quality System regulation. Each chapter addresses a section of the regulation, consisting of a restatement of the relevant section, a discussion of the requirements of that section, and a review of current industry practice.

The text draws on the collective wisdom of the foremost experts on the regulation from all related disciplines, including FDA, corporate representatives, and leading industry consultants. *The Quality System Compendium* is the result of more than a year of collaboration and consensus-building.

As part of AAMI's commitment to leadership in medical device quality systems, the compendium also serves as the basis for AAMI's intensive course on *GMP Requirements & Industry Practice*. As FDA policies evolve and as more experience is gained with the Quality System regulation, the text and the course will be refined and revised.

The Association for the Advancement of Medical Instrumentation wishes to gratefully acknowledge the immeasurable contributions of Wm. Fred Hooten, Hogan & Hartson; Edward McDonnell, Biometric Research Institute, Inc.; and Susan C. Reilly, Medical Device Consultants, Inc. Mr. Hooten and Mr. McDonnell coordinated the initial development of *The Quality System Compendium*, as well as the planning of the AAMI educational program, *GMP Requirements & Industry Practice*. Ms. Reilly authored sections of the compendium and served as the technical editor for the final text, ensuring its accuracy, clarity, and consistency with respect to FDA's final Quality System regulation.

The Association also wishes to express its deepest appreciation to the expert authors of the compendium, who drafted the original chapters, reviewed subsequent revisions, and offered critiques of their respective chapters as well as other portions of the volume:

Cheryl Boyce, Boyce Regulatory & Quality Consulting
Vera A. Buffaloe, Medical Device Consultant
William J. Feingold, Spektra Management Consultants, Inc.
Chris Flahive, Chris Flahive Associates
Wm. Fred Hooten, Hogan & Hartson
John J. Malloy, Malloy and Associates, Inc.
Edward McDonnell, Biometric Research Institute, Inc.
Dale McMillen, GMP Institute
Jane Moffitt, Consultant
Philip E. Nickerson, Consultant
Daniel P. Olivier, Computer Applications Specialists
Virginia Perry, Perry-D'Amico and Associates
Susan C. Reilly, Medical Device Consultants, Inc.
James W. Sandberg, Protocol Systems, Inc.
John Sawyer, OEC Medical Systems
Patricia B. Shrader, Becton-Dickinson and Company
Anita Thibeault, Anita Thibeault and Associates
William R. Trilsch, William Trilsch and Associates

The Association is also very grateful for the contributions of the members of the AAMI GMP Steering Committee and AAMI GMP Education and Training Committee, including the participation of FDA personnel. Both committees volunteered their time and considerable expertise for more than a year to develop AAMI's educational program on the Quality System regulation.

The **AAMI GMP Steering Committee** has the following members:

Cochairs: Wm. Fred Hooten, Edward McDonnell, Eileen Smith

Members: Joseph S. Arcarese, The Food and Drug Law Institute
Robert G. Britain, National Electrical Manufacturers Association
William J. Feingold, Spektra Management Consultants, Inc.
Wm. Fred Hooten, Hogan & Hartson
Bernard Liebler, Health Industry Manufacturers Association
David M. Link, ExperTech Associates
Burton I. Love, Regulatory Affairs Professionals Society
Edward McDonnell, Biometric Research Institute, Inc.
Eileen Smith, Association for the Advancement of Medical Instrumentation
Pamela Wojtowicz, Regulatory Affairs Professionals Society

The **AAMI GMP Education and Training Committee** has the following members:

Cochairs: Wm. Fred Hooten, Edward McDonnell, Eileen Smith

Members: Joseph S. Arcarese, The Food and Drug Law Institute
Link Bonforte, Regulatory Affairs Professionals Society
Cheryl Boyce, Boyce Regulatory & Quality Consulting
Robert G. Britain, National Electrical Manufacturers Association
Vera A. Buffaloe, Medical Device Consultant
David L. Chesney, Kemper-Masterson, Inc.
Richard J. DeRisio, Sorin Biomedical, Inc.
William J. Feingold, Spektra Management Consultants, Inc.
Chris Flahive, Chris Flahive Associates
Wm. Fred Hooten, Hogan & Hartson
Bernard Liebler, Health Industry Manufacturers Association
David M. Link, ExperTech Associates
John J. Malloy, Malloy and Associates, Inc.
Edward McDonnell, Biometric Research Institute, Inc.
Dale McMillen, GMP Institute
Jane Moffitt, Consultant
Philip E. Nickerson, Consultant
Daniel P. Olivier, Computer Applications Specialists
Virginia Perry, Perry-D'Amico and Associates
Frank Pokrop, Abbott Laboratories
Robert Reich, Pharmaceutical Systems, Inc.
Susan C. Reilly, Medical Device Consultants, Inc.
Beth Rice, Regulatory Resources
James W. Sandberg, Protocol Systems, Inc.
John Sawyer, OEC Medical Systems
Denise Schottler, Optical Systems, Inc.
Patricia B. Shrader, Becton-Dickinson and Company
Eileen Smith, Association for the Advancement of Medical Instrumentation

AAMI GMP Education and Training Committee *(continued)*

Members: William P. Taylor, Becton-Dickinson and Company
Linda K. Temple, Regulatory Affairs Professionals Society
Anita Thibeault, Anita Thibeault and Associates
William R. Trilsch, William Trilsch and Associates
Frank Twardochleb, C.L. McIntosh and Associates, Inc.
Gale E. Van Buskirk, RegTech, Ltd.

Finally, AAMI acknowledges the assistance of Kathy Warye, the former AAMI staff member who initially organized and coordinated the project, and Judith A. Veale, who edited the text.

CHAPTER 1. INTRODUCTION

In the October 7, 1996, issue of the *Federal Register*, the Food and Drug Administration (FDA) published as a final rule the Quality System regulation that supersedes the Good Manufacturing Practice (GMP) regulation promulgated in 1978. The final rule culminated a revision process undertaken by FDA, under the authority of the Safe Medical Devices Act (SMDA) of 1990, to amend the original GMP regulation to incorporate preproduction design controls and to implement other quality system requirements for consistency with ISO 13485, *Quality Systems -- Medical Devices -- Supplementary Requirements to ISO 9001*.

Recognizing the critical need for expertise in interpreting and applying the Quality System regulation, AAMI has developed an educational program for GMP consultants and corporate quality assurance and regulatory affairs professionals. The primary goals of the program are to establish a common body of knowledge on the Quality System regulation and to provide a series of educational courses that will be credible and beneficial to regulatory and quality professionals, medical device manufacturers, GMP consultants, and the FDA. It is envisioned that the program will ultimately benefit all those involved in medical device manufacturing by bringing greater uniformity and consistency to the interpretation and application of the medical device GMP requirements.

This compendium describes each of the requirements of the Quality System regulation. It begins with a regulatory overview and a general introduction to the Quality System regulation. The specific GMP requirements are grouped into eight major subject areas: general provisions, quality management, design, acceptance activities, production and process control, product control, monitoring and feedback, and documents and records. For each major section or subsection of the Quality System regulation, the requirement is quoted and discussed, and current industry practice is described. A comprehensive list of applicable references is provided in the appendix.

This compendium embodies the core body of knowledge upon which the AAMI educational program, "GMP Requirements & Industry Practice," is based. It is expected that the compendium will be revised as FDA policy evolves and as more experience is gained with the Quality System regulation. It is also expected that the compendium will be supplemented by materials provided at AAMI GMP educational courses.

CHAPTER 2. ABBREVIATIONS AND ACRONYMS USED IN THIS COMPENDIUM

AAMI: Association for the Advancement of Medical Instrumentation

ANSI: American National Standards Institute

ASQC: American Society for Quality Control

ASTM: American Society for Testing and Materials

ATE: automated test equipment

CDRH: Center for Devices and Radiological Health

CEO: chief executive officer

CNC: computerized numerical control

DCN: document change notice

DCO: document change order

DCR: document change request

DHF: design history file

DHR: device history record

DMR: device master record

DSMA: Division of Small Manufacturers Assistance

ECN: engineering change notice

ECO: engineering change order

ECR: engineering change request

EIR: establishment inspection report

EPA: Environmental Protection Agency

ESD: Electrostatic discharge

FDA: Food and Drug Administration

FDCA: Federal Food, Drug, and Cosmetic Act

FIFO: first in, first out

FOI: Freedom of Information

FMEA: failure modes and effects analysis

FTA: fault tree analysis

GLP: good laboratory practice

GMP: good manufacturing practice

HEPA: high-efficiency particulate air

HR: human resources

HVAC: heating, ventilation, and air conditioning

IDE: investigational device exemption

IEC: International Electrotechnical Commission

IEEE: Institute of Electrical and Electronic Engineers

ISO: International Organization for Standardization

MDR: medical device report

MRB: material review board

MRC: material review committee

NIST: National Institute of Standards and Technology

ODE: Office of Device Evaluation

ORA: Office of Regulatory Affairs

OSHA: Occupational Safety and Health Administration

PCB: printed circuit board

PDP: product development protocol

PERT: program evaluation and review technique

PMA: premarket approval

PMAA: premarket approval application

QA: quality assurance

QSR: quality system record

R&D: research and development

SMDA: Safe Medical Devices Act of 1990

SOP: standard operating procedure

TAPPI: Technical Association of the Paper and Pulp Industry

USP: U.S. Pharmacopeia

REGULATORY OVERVIEW

CHAPTER 3. ORGANIZATION AND REGULATORY STRATEGIES OF THE FDA

This chapter covers the following topics: the organization of FDA, with emphasis on the medical device enforcement staff; the actions that FDA can take to enforce the law; the types of inspections permitted under the law; recent trends in enforcement activities; and, compliance programs.

Organization of the FDA

The Food and Drug Administration is responsible for ensuring that

a) foods are safe, wholesome, and sanitary; human and veterinary drugs, biological products, and medical devices are safe and effective; cosmetics are safe; and electronic products that emit radiation are safe;

b) regulated products are honestly, accurately, and informatively represented;

c) regulated products are in compliance with the law and FDA regulations; noncompliance is identified and corrected; and, any unsafe or unlawful products are removed from the marketplace.

General Organization

The agency is headed by a presidentially appointed and Senate-confirmed Commissioner and by several civil service Deputy Commissioners, including the Deputy Commissioner for Operations. There are 10 Associate Commissioners, among whom is the Associate Commissioner for Regulatory Affairs; and there are six centers at headquarters that regulate substantive product areas, such as the Center for Devices and Radiological Health (CDRH). The field organization consists of 5 regional field offices, 21 district offices, and 137 resident inspection posts.

Figure 1 is an overall organizational chart of the agency. Of most direct interest to GMP professionals are the activities of FDA's Office of Regulatory Affairs (ORA) (figure 2) and Center for Devices and Radiological Health (figure 3). The bulk of FDA's enforcement activity originates from the district offices and resident inspection posts (figure 4). The enforcement functions of the field offices apply to all FDA-regulated product areas. The agency's device enforcement activities are guided by CDRH policies and procedures and implemented by the field offices.

Center for Devices and Radiological Health

The CDRH is responsible for ensuring the safety and effectiveness of medical devices and eliminating unnecessary human exposure to man-made radiation from medical, occupational, and consumer-product sources. Specifically, CDRH

a) reviews and evaluates medical device premarket approval applications (PMAAs), product

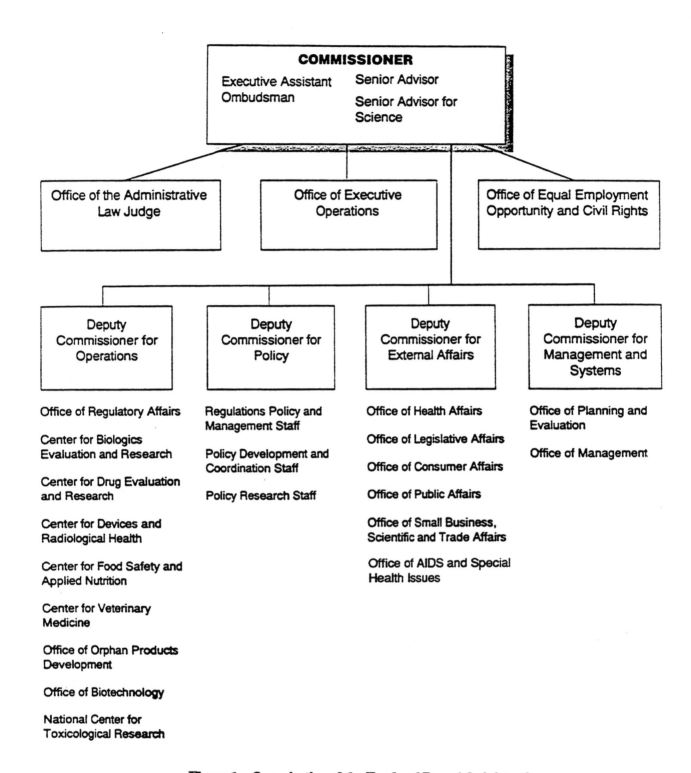

Figure 1 – Organization of the Food and Drug Administration

development protocols (PDPs), requests for investigational device exemptions (IDEs), and 510(k) premarket notifications;

b) collects information about injuries and other experiences in the use of medical devices and radiation-emitting electronic products and uses this information in Center activities;

c) develops, promulgates, and enforces GMP regulations and performance standards for radiation-emitting electronic products and medical devices;

d) monitors compliance and surveillance programs for medical devices and radiation-emitting electronic products; and,

e) provides technical and other nonfinancial assistance to small medical device manufacturers.

Personnel

Field personnel include consumer safety officers, who are employed in both the compliance and investigation branches of the district offices. In the investigation branch, they are called investigators; in the compliance branch, they are called compliance officers. Some investigators are trained to conduct inspections of all product areas that FDA regulates, but most receive specialized training in particular product areas (e.g., medical devices, drugs, foods) and/or technologies (e.g., software-controlled devices). Compliance officers generally are more experienced than investigators and analysts. District offices also employ consumer safety inspectors; and FDA has the authority to hire up to 95 criminal investigators.

Office of Regulatory Affairs

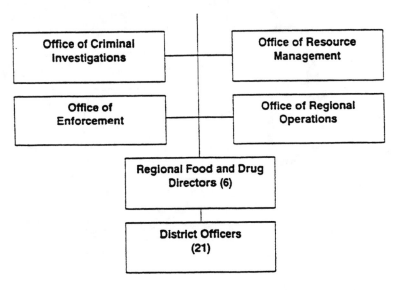

Figure 2 – Organization of FDA's Office of Regulatory Affairs

Center for Devices and Radiological Health

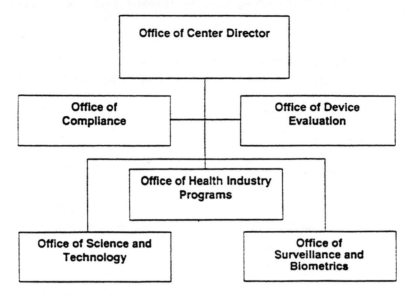

Figure 3 – Organization of FDA's Center for Devices and Radiological Health

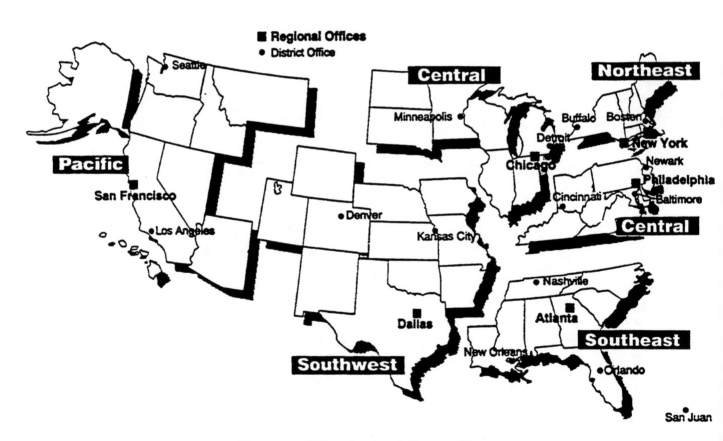

Figure 4 – FDA regional and district offices

Compliance Programs

The FDA uses the Compliance Program Manual as a convenient and organized system for issuing and filing written program plans and instructions for FDA field operations. The present system was inaugurated in October 1974; it is revised occasionally to make the programs more concise.

The Center for Devices and Radiological Health and the Office of Regulatory Affairs collaborate in the development and preparation of compliance programs with regard to strategy, objectives, timetables, and goals. Typically, CDRH drafts a program subject to ORA review and input. The completed compliance program contains FDA's inspectional priorities. The field work plan, which is a separate document issued to each FDA district office, identifies how many inspections the district must complete in each compliance program.

Compliance programs serve the following purposes:

a) They provide uniform guidance and specific instructions for gathering and presenting evidence needed to support the various FDA regulatory enforcement initiatives.

b) They provide guidance to field investigators and laboratory personnel for gathering product or industry information within a specific timeframe to determine the existence or extent of a problem.

c) They provide a mechanism by which Centers can accumulate data on known problems to determine long-range trends on a statistical basis.

Each compliance program is organized into seven parts:

Part I (Background) presents a brief description of the historical data, the rationale for the program, and relevant legal authorities.

Part II (Implementation) sets forth the specific objectives of the program and brief program management instructions.

Part III (Inspectional) describes the inspectional operations that the field is expected to carry out, with special attention to field reporting requirements.

Part IV (Analytical) specifies the analyzing laboratories and analyses to be performed, as well as any special reporting requirements.

Part V (Regulatory/Administrative Strategy) provides direction and guidance to the field on what to do when the inspection documents deficiencies or violations. It describes the types of violations that warrant regulatory follow-up and what regulatory action the field should take.

Part VI (References, Attachments, and Contacts) lists supplemental information important to understanding how the program is to work.

Part VII (Center Responsibilities) provides specific instructions to the appropriate Center, identifying the type of evaluation that the Center must complete at the end of the program.

Compliance programs are available from FDA's Division of Small Manufacturers Assistance (DSMA) and are one of the best sources for understanding FDA's regulatory priorities. The inspectional instructions describe the nature and type of inspection to be conducted. Quality professionals should carefully review the questions that FDA investigators will ask so that their firms will be able to respond to inspection inquiries. Perhaps the most important section of a compliance program is Part V, which contains specific information on regulatory strategy, including philosophy on voluntary compliance, regulatory opinions, regulatory options, special considerations, mitigating circumstances, and special case guidance on what to do if certain situations are encountered. District compliance officers use Part V when deciding if regulatory attention is warranted. Regulatory professionals need to be familiar with this section.

Presently, there are 18 medical device compliance programs referenced in the ORA field work plan:

7382.001	Inspection of Manufacturers of Laser Products
7382.002	Field Implementation of the Sunlamp and Sunlamp Products
7382.003	Field Compliance Testing of Diagnostic (Medical X-Ray) Equipment
7382.004	Field Compliance Testing of Cabinet X-Ray Equipment
7382.006	Compliance Testing of Electronic Products at WEAC
7382.006G	WEAC Testing of Medical Devices for Conformance to Voluntary Standards
7382.007	Imported Electronic Products
7382007A	Imported Noncertified Radiation-Emitting Electronic Products
7382.008	Monitoring Devices of Foreign Origin -- Import
7382.009	Suspected Deceptive and Fraudulent Devices
7382.010	Medical Device Problem Reporting
7382.011	Enforcement of the Medical Device Reporting (MDR) Regulation
7382.013	Conformance Assessment of Devices to Product Specifications
7382.830	**Inspection of Medical Device Manufacturers**
7382.830A	Sterilization of Medical Devices
7382.830B	Contract Sterilizers
7383.001	Medical Device Premarket Approval and Post Market Inspection
7383.003	510(k) Premarket Approval Inspections

Compliance Program 7382.830, *Inspection of Medical Device Manufacturers,* is the largest program (in terms of resources), and it contains valuable information on how FDA measures compliance with the device GMP requirements.

Inspections

The Food and Drug Administration is mandated by law to inspect manufacturers of class II and class III devices at least once every 2 years. In addition, all PMAA approvals and all 510(k) clearances of class III devices are contingent upon completion of a satisfactory facility inspection. Inspections may also be made in connection with surveys conducted prior to issuing new regulations; audits of clinical investigators; and recalls, enforcement actions, serious complaints, or significant medical device reports (MDRs). When warning letters or other significant compliance issues arise as the result of an inspection, a reinspection is likely within 6 months. The FDA also conducts foreign inspections of manufacturers that distribute FDA-regulated products in the United States.

FDA Enforcement Authorities

If FDA determines that a manufacturer is in violation of the Federal Food, Drug, and Cosmetic Act (FDCA) or accompanying regulations, the agency may take the following enforcement or administrative actions:

a) warning letter (telling a company to notify FDA of the corrective action it plans to take within 15 days);

b) order to repair, replace, or refund with respect to certain devices;

c) notification to users or the public of an unreasonable risk of substantial harm to the public health;

d) PMAA withdrawal;

e) prohibition of import of devices made outside the United States;

f) device seizure;

g) injunction (preventing the manufacture and distribution of a device); and,

h) criminal prosecution of a company and/or responsible individuals.

The Safe Medical Devices Act of 1990 (SMDA) added provisions that enable FDA to

a) require a company to notify FDA of all corrections and withdrawals;

b) recall devices after an informal hearing and notify individuals subject to the risk presented by the device;

c) suspend a PMAA after an opportunity for an informal hearing;

d) order the cessation of shipment and distribution of devices prior to a hearing; and,

e) impose civil penalties in a proceeding before an administrative law judge up to a maximum of $15,000 per violation, not to exceed $1 million for all such violations, against individuals and companies.

Recent years have seen a streamlining of Headquarters' review of enforcement actions.

Warning Letters

In most cases, warning letters are issued directly by the district directors, according to guidance provided in compliance programs issued by each Center. In some cases, where technical evaluation of complex scientific/medical data is required, headquarters concurrence is necessary. Such letters do not commit FDA to enforcement action but do warn that the lack of prompt corrective action may result in enforcement action. Warning letters are issued only for violations of significance and generally require a response from the manufacturer within 15 working days. Warning letters are on public display at FDA's Freedom of Information (FOI) office.

"Direct Reference Authority"

In some instances, through "Direct Reference Authority," FDA has empowered the field to take action with less review by headquarters. Direct Reference Authority is applicable to marketing a class III device without required premarket review; marketing surgical gloves that do not meet certain criteria; and marketing misbranded electrical muscle stimulators.

Foreign Inspections

The FDA has significantly increased the number of foreign inspections that it conducts. Foreign companies that fail to meet GMP requirements are subject to warning letters and to warning letters with import detention orders that prohibit entry of their devices into the United States until violations are corrected.

510(k) Modifications

In recent years, FDA has focused attention on modifications to devices for which new 510(k) premarket notifications have not been filed, with the result that companies have been requested to cease marketing and/or file new 510(k) submissions.

Criminal Prosecution

Through new rules, it is now simpler and faster for FDA to refer criminal cases to the Department of Justice.

Traditional Enforcement Chain of Command

In the "bottom-up" scenario, a device-related recommendation proceeds from an investigator or compliance officer to the director of the district office and then to CDRH for review by the Office of

Compliance and, in some cases, the Center director. Concurrence in the action by the Office of the Chief Counsel and the Associate Commissioner for Regulatory Affairs may also be required (e.g., in the case of seizures). In criminal cases and other court actions, the matter is referred to the Department of Justice. Cases may be tried by FDA attorneys, in conjunction with lawyers from Justice serving in the local U.S. Attorney's Office.

In the "top-down" scenario, a device-related recommendation may originate in CDRH, which can direct the districts to pursue various enforcement actions. These actions often require subsequent review at headquarters.

CHAPTER 4. HISTORY OF DEVELOPMENT OF THE QUALITY SYSTEM REGULATION

The Quality System regulation, published by FDA as a final rule on October 7, 1996, revises the 1978 GMP regulation by replacing quality assurance (QA) program requirements with quality system requirements that include new provisions concerning the design, purchasing, and servicing of medical devices. The current regulation also codifies FDA's interpretation of the 1978 GMP regulation in regard to record-keeping requirements for device failure and complaint investigations, and it clarifies the requirements for process validation, product change control, and the collection and evaluation of quality data. As part of the revision process, FDA has attempted to harmonize the device Quality System regulation with ISO 13485, *Quality systems -- Medical devices -- Supplementary requirements to ISO 9001*.

The 1978 GMP Regulation

The GMP requirements for medical devices (21 CFR Part 820) were first authorized by the Medical Device Amendments of 1976 (section 520[f]) of the Federal Food, Drug, and Cosmetic Act (21 U.S.C. 360j[f]). In response to the new authority provided by section 520(f), FDA issued final regulations in the *Federal Register* of July 21, 1978 (43 FR 31508), prescribing GMP requirements for the methods used in, and the facilities and controls used for, the manufacture, packing, storage, and installation of medical devices. This regulation became effective on December 18, 1978, and is codified under part 820.

In drafting the 1978 regulation, FDA recognized that the medical device industry consists of manufacturers whose devices and manufacturing processes differ significantly. Therefore, the GMP regulation was designed to specify general requirements in areas of concern applicable to all manufacturers, as well as additional requirements for high-risk devices, which were termed "critical devices." This two-tier approach was intended to prevent excessive regulation of the device industry. Each manufacturer was expected to supply the details of an appropriate GMP program by developing for the manufacture of each device a detailed set of procedures implementing the GMP regulation. The agency would then examine these procedures to determine whether a manufacturer was complying with the regulation. This flexible, umbrella GMP philosophy is carried over into the current Quality System regulation.

The Revision Process

Until the promulgation of the Quality System regulation, the medical device GMP requirements had not been revised since 1978, except for editorial changes to update organizational references and revisions to the list of critical devices that was included in the preamble to the final 1978 regulation. The Quality System regulation is the result of a revision effort begun in 1990.

Due to a number of studies and recall evaluations indicating that a significant number of device failures were due to design defects,* FDA began promoting the addition of design controls to the GMP regulation. In response, industry took a common position that FDA did not have the authority to add design controls to the regulation. This difference of opinion between FDA and the industry became a nonissue on November 28, 1990, when Congress passed the Safe Medical Devices Act of 1990 (SMDA). The SMDA amended section 520(f) of the FDCA, providing FDA with the authority to add preproduction design controls to the GMP regulation.

The SMDA also included a new section 803, which encourages FDA to work with foreign countries toward mutual recognition of GMP and other regulations. For a number of years previously, FDA had already been working with the European Community, Canada, Australia, and Japan in an effort to harmonize requirements. The revision of the GMP regulation, including the design controls authorized by the SMDA, allows the regulation to be consistent, where feasible, with the requirements contained in applicable international standards, specifically ISO 9001:1994, *Quality systems: Model for quality assurance in design, development, production, installation, and servicing*, and ISO 13485, *Quality systems -- Medical devices -- Supplementary requirements to ISO 9001*.

An advanced notice of proposed rulemaking appeared in the *Federal Register* on June 15, 1990. This notice announced FDA's intent to revise the GMP regulation. On November 30, 1990, a notice of availability of a document, "Medical Devices: Current Good Manufacturing Practices (CGMP) Regulations Document; Suggested Changes; Availability," appeared in the *Federal Register*.

The first proposed rule revising the GMP requirements was published in the November 23, 1993, issue of the *Federal Register*. This proposal consisted basically of the ISO requirements, plus those requirements of the 1978 regulation that are not part of ISO 13485. Approximately 280 separate individuals or groups commented on this proposal.

The agency announced the second proposal in a July 1995 "Notice of Availability of a Working Draft of the CGMP Final Rule." Approximately 175 separate individuals or groups commented on the draft. Shortly after the release of the July 1995 Working Draft, FDA held an open public meeting and a GMP Advisory Committee meeting to solicit public comment.

Principal Differences Between the 1978 GMP Regulation and the Quality System Regulation

As mentioned previously, the 1978 GMP regulation imposed additional requirements on "critical devices," which were defined as devices that are intended for surgical implant into the body or devices intended to support or sustain life and whose failure to perform when properly used according to the labeling can be reasonably expected to result in significant injury to the user. The term "critical device" has been eliminated in the Quality System regulation; however, the regulation still

---

*Specifically, FDA's January 1990 publication, *Device Recalls: A Study of Quality Problems* (HHS Publication FD 90-4235), and the 1990 Department of Health and Human Services Inspector General's study, *FDA Medical Device Regulation from Premarket Review to Recall*.

allows manufacturers the flexibility to determine the amount or degree of action necessary commensurate with the risk associated with the product.

The Quality System regulation incorporates new requirements for preproduction design control and supplier control. Servicing controls for manufacturers also have been added. Although inherent in the 1978 GMP regulation, specific language for management responsibilities, process validation, corrective and preventive action, quality system records, and statistical techniques is explicit in the Quality System regulation.

GENERAL PROVISIONS OF THE QUALITY SYSTEM REGULATION

CHAPTER 5. GENERAL PROVISIONS (SUBPART A)

820.1 SCOPE

820.1(a) APPLICABILITY

820.1 Scope

(a) Applicability

(1) Current good manufacturing practice (CGMP) requirements are set forth in this quality system regulation. The requirements in this part govern the methods used in, and the facilities and controls used for, the design, manufacture, packaging, labeling, storage, installation, and servicing of all finished devices intended for human use. The requirements in this part are intended to ensure that finished devices will be safe and effective and otherwise in compliance with the Federal Food, Drug, and Cosmetic Act (the act). This part establishes basic requirements applicable to manufacturers of finished medical devices. If a manufacturer engages in only some operations subject to the requirements in this part, and not in others, that manufacturer need only comply with those requirements applicable to the operations in which it is engaged. With respect to class I devices, design controls apply only to those devices listed in [section] 820.30(a)(2). This regulation does not apply to manufacturers of components or parts of finished devices, but such manufacturers are encouraged to use appropriate provisions of this regulation as guidance. Manufacturers of human blood and blood components are not subject to this part, but are subject to part 606 of this chapter.

(2) The provisions of this part shall be applicable to any finished device as defined in this part, intended for human use, that is manufactured, imported, or offered for import in any State or Territory of the United States, the District of Columbia, or the Commonwealth of Puerto Rico.

(3) In this regulation the term "where appropriate" is used several times. When a requirement is qualified by "where appropriate," it is deemed to be "appropriate" unless the manufacturer can document justification otherwise. A requirement is "appropriate" if nonimplementation could reasonably be expected to result in the product not meeting its specified requirements or the manufacturer not being able to carry out any necessary corrective action.

Discussion: The requirements of the Quality System regulation are generally harmonized with current international quality standards for medical devices. The regulation provides an outline of basic requirements for a manufacturer to use when establishing a quality system.

The GMP requirements of the Quality System regulation apply to manufacturers of finished medical devices that are intended for human use. Manufacturers of human blood and blood components are not subject to 21 CFR 820, but rather to 21 CFR 606, "Current Good Manufacturing Practice for Blood and Blood Components." Component manufacturers are not required to comply with the regulation, but are encouraged to use the regulation as a guideline.

820.1(b) LIMITATIONS

*820.1(b) **Limitations.** The quality system regulation in this part supplements regulations in other parts of this chapter except where explicitly stated otherwise. In the event that it is impossible to comply with all applicable regulations, both in this part and in other parts of this chapter, the regulations specifically applicable to the device in question shall supersede any other generally applicable requirements.*

Discussion: The Quality System regulation applies to all medical devices unless specifically stated otherwise in other 21 CFR regulations that apply to medical devices. For example, the classification regulations exempt certain class I devices from GMP requirements. If it is impossible to comply with all of the applicable regulations, because of conflicting requirements, the regulation that is specifically applicable to the device in question takes precedence.

820.1(c) AUTHORITY

*820.1(c) **Authority.** Part 820 is established and promulgated under authority of sections 501, 502, 510, 513, 514, 515, 518, 519, 520, 522, 701, 704, 801, 803 of the act (21 U.S.C. 351, 352, 360, 360c, 360d, 360e, 360h, 360i, 360j, 360l, 371, 374, 381, 383). The failure to comply with any applicable provision in this part renders the device adulterated under section 501(h) of the act. Such a device, as well as the person responsible for the failure to comply, is subject to regulatory action under sections 301, 302, 303, 304, and 801 of the act.*

Discussion: This section states the legal authority under which the GMP requirements are written. For example, part 519 provides FDA with the authority to require the records mandated by the Quality System regulation. Also, this section defines the consequences of failing to comply with the regulation. Failure to comply with *any* GMP requirement may render the device adulterated and subject to the adulteration penalties of the act.

820.1(d) FOREIGN MANUFACTURERS

*820.1(d) **Foreign manufacturers.** If a manufacturer who offers devices for import into the United States refuses to permit or allow the completion of a Food and Drug Administration (FDA) inspection of the foreign facility for the purpose of determining compliance with this part, it shall appear for purposes of section 801 (a) of the act, that the methods used in, and the facilities and controls used for, the design, manufacture, packaging, labeling, storage, installation, or servicing of any devices produced at such facility that are offered for import into the United States do not conform to the requirements of section 520(f) of the act and this part and that the devices manufactured at that facility are adulterated under section 501(h) of the act.*

Discussion: The FDA has no authority outside the United States and must obtain permission from the manufacturers to audit foreign establishments. If a foreign manufacturer refuses to allow an FDA audit, the manufacturer's products will be considered adulterated and will not be allowed to be distributed in the United States. This requirement resulted from refusals by certain foreign manufacturers to allow FDA inspections and from delays in allowing such inspections.

820.1(e) EXEMPTIONS OR VARIANCES

820.1(e) Exemptions or variances. (1) Any person who wishes to petition for an exemption or variance from any device quality system requirement is subject to the requirements of section 520(f)(2) of the act. Petitions for an exemption or variance shall be submitted according to the procedures set forth in [section] 10.30 of this chapter, the FDA's administrative procedures. Guidance is available from the Center for Devices and Radiological Health, Division of Small Manufacturers Assistance, (HFZ-220), 1350 Piccard Dr., Rockville, MD 20850, U.S.A., telephone 1-800-638-2041 or 1-301-443-6597, FAX 301-443-8818.

(2) FDA may initiate and grant a variance from any device quality system requirement when the agency determines that such variance is in the best interest of the public health. Such variance will remain in effect only so long as there remains a public need for the device and the device would not likely be made sufficiently available without the variance.

Discussion: Anyone may petition for an exemption or variance from all or part of the Quality System regulation and may even propose entirely different quality systems. An exemption means that a manufacturer is not required to comply. A variance is permission to substitute a control for one required by the regulation. To date, FDA has received fewer than 100 petitions for variances and exemptions. All of those approved have been petitions for removal from the critical device list. Generally, because of the flexibility of this regulation, exemptions and variances have not been justified.

Guidelines for the submission of petitions for exemptions or variances are available from FDA's Division of Small Manufacturers Assistance. The agency may not process a petition while an FDA investigation is ongoing.

820.3 DEFINITIONS

820.3(a) Act means the Federal Food, Drug, and Cosmetic Act, as amended (secs. 201-903, 52 Stat. 1040 et seq., as amended (21 U.S.C. 321-394)). All definitions in section 201 of the act shall apply to these regulations.

Discussion: Section 201 of the act contains a number of definitions, including the definition of "device":

"an instrument, apparatus, implement, machine, contrivance, implant, in vitro reagent, or other similar or related article, including any component, part, or accessory, which is --

"(1) recognized in the official National Formulary, or the United States Pharmacopoeia, or any supplement to them,

"(2) intended for use in the diagnosis of disease or other conditions, or in the cure, mitigation, treatment, or prevention of disease, in man or other animals, or

"(3) intended to affect the structure or any function of the body of man or other animals, and

"which does not achieve its primary intended purposes through chemical action within or on the body of man or other animals and which is not dependent upon being metabolized for the achievement of its primary intended purposes."

820.3(b) Complaint means any written, electronic, or oral communication that alleges deficiencies related to the identity, quality, durability, reliability, safety, effectiveness, or performance of a device after it is released for distribution.

Discussion: A complaint can be from any source, but is only considered to be a complaint when the communication alleges a deficiency related to the characteristics identified above. However, there is one condition defined in the regulation that must be considered to be a complaint, even if there are no allegations of a deficiency: the requirement under section 820.200(a) that all events meeting the medical device reporting (MDR) criteria must be considered to be and investigated as complaints as per section 820.198. However, the fact that an event may not meet the complaint definition does not mean that it should not be investigated and corrective action taken, when necessary. All quality problems must be identified, evaluated, and resolved under section 820.100, "Corrective and preventive action."

820.3(c) Component means any raw material, substance, piece, part, software, firmware, labeling, or assembly which is intended to be included as part of the finished, packaged, and labeled device.

Discussion: All materials, as specified in this definition, are subject to component controls. These controls include the requirements of section 820.80(b), "Receiving acceptance activities."

820.3(d) Control number means any distinctive symbols, such as a distinctive combination of letters or numbers, or both, from which the history of the manufacturing, packaging, labeling, and distribution of a unit, lot, or batch of finished devices can be determined.

Discussion: When traceability is required, the manufacturer's system and methods must ensure that a history of the device can be reproduced, to the degree necessary, to allow the investigation of quality problems, effective recalls, and corrective action. The level of detail required should be based on the nature, complexity, and use of the finished device.

820.3(e) Design history file (DHF) means a compilation of records which describes the design history of a finished device.

Discussion: The "design history file" (DHF) is intended to act as a repository for the data necessary to provide evidence that the design plan was followed. The file must contain or reference the records necessary to show that the design plan and applicable design control requirements were met. The DHF for each type of device developed should include, for example, the design and development plan, design specifications, design review results, design verification results, and design validation results.

820.3(f) Design input means the physical and performance requirements of a device that are used as a basis for device design.

Discussion: "Design input" includes information obtained on needs and requirements, such as intended use, performance, safety, user interface, compatibility, reliability, labeling, and packaging. Input requirements, translated into preliminary design specifications, should be established in measurable terms, including acceptable ranges and limits.

820.3(g) Design output means the results of a design effort at each design phase and at the end of the total design effort. The finished design output is the basis for the device master record. The total finished design output consists of the device, its packaging and labeling, and the device master record.

Discussion: Total "design output" is the results of each design phase. Design output should meet design input requirements, as confirmed through design validation and verification and ensured during design review. Design output includes the specifications, blueprints, test procedures, environmental requirements, and so forth that are finalized at the end of the design process and translated into manufacturing specifications, methods, and procedures. Final design output includes the device, its packaging and labeling, and the device master record (DMR).

820.3(h) Design review means a documented, comprehensive, systematic examination of a design to evaluate the adequacy of the design requirements, to evaluate the capability of the design to meet these requirements, and to identify problems.

Discussion: Each design review must be comprehensive for the design phase being reviewed. All aspects of the design process should be reviewed when the design is transferred.

*820.3(i) **Device history record (DHR*** *means a compilation of records containing the production history of a finished device.*

Discussion: The DHR is a collection of records that objectively demonstrates that a device was made in accordance with its DMR.

*820.3(j) **Device master record (DMR)*** *means a compilation of records containing the procedures and specifications for a finished device.*

Discussion: The types and extent of records that make up a manufacturer's DMR vary greatly. Key elements that a DMR must contain include device specifications; component specifications; product process specifications; quality assurance procedures and specifications; packaging and labeling specifications and methods; and installation, maintenance, and servicing procedures and methods.

*820.3(k) **Establish*** *means define, document (in writing or electronically), and implement.*

Discussion: Wherever the term appears, "establish" means that adequate written documentation, either hard-copy or electronic, must be in place. The term also means that the documents must be properly implemented.

*820.3(l) **Finished device*** *means any device or accessory to any device that is suitable for use or capable of functioning, whether or not it is packaged, labeled, or sterilized.*

Discussion: The Quality System regulation only applies to finished devices. Therefore, the definition of a finished device must be broad enough so that the quality system will be applied to the degree necessary to ensure that the device is safe and effective. The GMP requirements cannot be applied merely after a device is finished except for, say, sterilization, polishing, or testing. The definition states that a device must be "suitable for use or capable of functioning." "Capable of functioning" is not necessarily the same as "suitable for use." For example, an implantable pacemaker may be capable of functioning, but it is not suitable for use until it has been sterilized. However, it is considered a finished device for purposes of the Quality System regulation.

*820.3(m) **Lot or batch*** *means one or more components or finished devices that consist of a single type, model, class, size, composition, or software version that are manufactured under essentially the same conditions and that are intended to have uniform characteristics and quality within specified limits.*

Discussion: A lot or batch may comprise only one finished device or component. It is the manufacturer's responsibility to determine the appropriate size of a lot or batch, based on the device and associated manufacturing processes.

820.3(n) Management with executive responsibility *means those senior employees of a manufacturer who have the authority to establish or make changes to the manufacturer's quality policy and quality system.*

Discussion: The term "management with executive responsibility" is intended to apply only to management that has the *authority* to bring about change in the quality system and in the management of that system. "Management with executive responsibility" may be the chief executive officer (CEO), or the CEO may delegate the authority to other top-level executives to carry out the requirements of 21 CFR 820.20, "Management responsibility." Upper management may not delegate the responsibility for ensuring that the requirements are met.

820.3(o) Manufacturer *means any person who designs, manufactures, fabricates, assembles, or processes a finished device. Manufacturer includes but is not limited to those who perform the functions of contract sterilization, installation, relabeling, remanufacturing, repacking, or specification development, and initial distributors of foreign entities performing these functions.*

Discussion: Although FDA believes that persons who perform servicing and refurbishing activities outside the control of the original equipment manufacturer meet the definition of "manufacturer," the terms "servicer" and "refurbisher" are not included in the Quality System regulation. The FDA will address the application of GMP requirements to these functions in a separate rulemaking.

"Remanufacturer" is included in this definition because remanufacturing changes a finished device's specifications or intended use. Contract sterilizers, installers, specification developers, repackagers, relabelers, and initial distributors that perform one or more of the functions described in the definition are also considered manufacturers because these activities may have an effect on the safety and effectiveness of the device.

820.3(p) Manufacturing material *means any material or substance used in or used to facilitate the manufacturing process, a concomitant constituent, or a byproduct constituent produced during the manufacturing process, which is present in or on the finished device as a residue or impurity not by design or intent of the manufacturer.*

Discussion: "Concomitant constituent" is included in this definition as a result of FDA's experiences with medical gloves and is intended to address materials such as natural rubber latex, which may contain naturally occurring allergenic proteins that should be reduced or removed to a level at which they do not adversely affect the safety of the finished product.

820.3(q) Nonconformity means the nonfulfillment of a specified requirement.

Discussion: The FDA emphasizes that a nonconformity may not always constitute a product defect or failure, but a product defect or failure is typically a nonconformity. This definition is applicable to product before or after distribution.

820.3(r) Product means components, manufacturing materials, in-process devices, finished devices, and returned devices.

Discussion: As used in the Quality System regulation, the term "product" is consistent with the definition given in ISO 8402:1994. It is intended to avoid repetition of "components, manufacturing materials, in-process devices, finished devices, and returned devices" throughout the regulation.

820.3(s) Quality means the totality of features and characteristics that bear on the ability of a device to satisfy fitness-for-use, including safety and performance.

Discussion: This definition is a compromise between the desire to harmonize with ISO 8402:1994 and the need to include safety and effectiveness as necessary elements of fitness for use.

820.3(t) Quality audit means a systematic, independent examination of a manufacturer's quality system that is performed at defined intervals and at sufficient frequency to determine whether both quality system activities and the results of such activities comply with quality system procedures, that these procedures are implemented effectively, and that these procedures are suitable to achieve quality system objectives.

Discussion: Quality audits may be conducted in phases. It is not necessary for each audit to address the entire quality system, provided that the manufacturer examines the entire system at defined, regular intervals. These intervals should be sufficient to detect, correct, and prevent major problems.

820.3(u) Quality policy means the overall intentions and direction of an organization with respect to quality, as established by management with executive responsibility.

Discussion: The definition of "quality policy" is compatible with the definition in ISO 8402:1994. This definition makes it clear that FDA requires the quality policy to be implemented and enforced by top management.

820.3(v) *Quality system means the organizational structure, responsibilities, procedures, processes, and resources for implementing quality management.*

Discussion: This definition is also compatible with the definition in ISO 8402:1994. "Quality management" refers to the overall management activities and functions that determine and implement the quality policy, objectives, and responsibilities.

820.3(w) *Remanufacturer means any person who processes, conditions, renovates, repackages, restores, or does any other act to a finished device that significantly changes the finished device's performance or safety specifications, or intended use.*

Discussion: Anyone who changes the specifications of a device is considered to be a manufacturer. The FDA has maintained this position for many years. This definition is consistent with 510(k) provisions and PMA application/supplement requirements.

820.3(x) *Rework means action taken on a nonconforming product so that it will fulfill the specified DMR requirements before it is released for distribution.*

Discussion: The definition of "rework" applies to devices or components prior to distribution and relates to the requirements of section 820.90(b)(2), "Nonconformity review and disposition." Rework should be performed according to specified DMR requirements.

820.3(y) *Specification means any requirement with which a product, process, service, or other activity must conform.*

Discussion: This definition applies to the documented requirements for a product, process, service, or other activity, as defined by the manufacturer.

820.3(z) *Validation means confirmation by examination and provision of objective evidence that the particular requirements for a specific intended use can be consistently fulfilled.*

Discussion: The FDA has adopted the ISO 8402:1994 definition of "validation." Validation ensures that user needs and intended uses can be met consistently.

820.3(z)(1) *Process validation means establishing by objective evidence that a process consistently produces a result or product meeting its predetermined specifications.*

Discussion: The definition of "process validation" is consistent with the definition of "validation" that appears in FDA's 1987 guidance document, *Guideline on General Principles of Process Validation*.

820.3(z)(2) **Design validation** *means establishing by objective evidence that device specifications conform with user needs and intended use(s).*

Discussion: Design validation ensures that the finished product meets the requirements for its intended use. Design validation follows successful design verification.

820.3(aa) **Verification** *means confirmation by examination and provision of objective evidence that specified requirements have been fulfilled.*

Discussion: The FDA has adopted the ISO 8402:1994 definition of "verification." Verification ensures that outputs for a particular device or activity meet the specified input requirements. Examples of verification are software module testing and prototype testing.

QUALITY MANAGEMENT

CHAPTER 6. QUALITY SYSTEM (SUBPART A)

820.5 QUALITY SYSTEM

The Requirement

820.5 Quality system. Each manufacturer shall establish and maintain a quality system that is appropriate for the specific medical device(s) designed or manufactured, and that meets the requirements of this part.

Discussion of the Requirement

The general requirements of section 820.5 are the basis on which the specific requirements of the Quality System regulation are built. Each manufacturer is required to design, implement, and maintain an appropriate quality system, including instructions and procedures, to meet the requirements of the regulation. By meeting the requirements of the Quality System regulation, the manufacturer is ensuring, as required by section 820.1, the safety and effectiveness of the particular device(s) produced.

CHAPTER 7. QUALITY SYSTEM REQUIREMENTS (SUBPART B)

820.20 MANAGEMENT RESPONSIBILITY

820.20(a) QUALITY POLICY

The Requirement

*820.20(a) **Quality policy.** Management with executive responsibility shall establish its policy and objectives for, and commitment to, quality. Management with executive responsibility shall ensure that the quality policy is understood, implemented, and maintained at all levels of the organization.*

Discussion of the Requirement

Section 820.3(u) of the regulation defines "quality policy" as "the overall quality intentions and direction of an organization with respect to quality, as formally expressed by management with executive responsibility." Section 820.3(n) defines "management with executive responsibility" as "those senior employees of a manufacturer who have the authority to establish or make changes to the manufacturer's quality policy and quality system."

This section of the regulation requires a manufacturer to establish a quality policy and objectives. Management with executive responsibility is required to define this policy and to communicate it to all employees. While the establishment of quality objectives, the development of methods and procedures based on these objectives, and the implementation of the quality system may be delegated, it is the responsibility of top management to establish the quality policy and ensure that it is followed.

The FDA believes that it is without question management's responsibility to ensure that employees understand the quality policy and objectives. Furthermore, FDA believes that understanding is a learning process achieved through education and reinforcement. Management with executive responsibility reinforces understanding of the quality policy by demonstrating a commitment to the quality system, visibly and actively, on a continuous basis.

Industry Practice

During the last decade, the medical device industry has become more sophisticated in implementing quality programs based both on internal and external factors. Internally, companies are faced with customers demanding quality products and services. Externally, competition has pressured companies to improve quality while controlling costs. Companies have established quality programs based on concepts such as Total Quality Management and Quality Leadership and on recognized quality standards such as the ISO 9000 series. Within these quality programs, establishing a quality policy is a requirement.

Management with executive responsibility sets the quality policy and attitude for the company, regardless of the size of the company. In addition, ensuring that the company quality policy is understood by all personnel involves formal education and training.

The following are some examples of quality policies:

Company A

"It is our Quality Policy to

a) strive to achieve total quality performance, by understanding who the Company's customers are and what their requirements are regarding product and services;

b) ensure, by internal quality audits and third party assessment, that the appropriate quality level is achieved, thus assuring that our goods and services are safe and effective for their intended use and that the specifications for these goods and services are consistently achieved;

c) continuously strive to improve the quality of the Company's products; and,

d) work at all times in the manner defined in the Company's documented Quality System, thus ensuring that the standards defined in 21 CFR 820 and ISO 9001 are being maintained."

Company B

"Our ongoing objective is to provide the most technologically advanced, high performance and high quality products, as well as the most advanced customer service. We are committed to meeting the needs of our worldwide customers, both internal and external to the company, and continuing to strive for excellence in everything we do as a company.

"The well-being of patients throughout the world depends on the performance of our products; therefore, quality and reliability are critical. It is essential that we do our utmost to ensure that quality is an integral part of every function of this company.

"Our Total Quality Program has been designed to provide an effective means of maximizing quality and assuring that manufactured products fulfill their intended purpose with regard to safety, performance, reliability, appearance, and customer satisfaction. The Vice President of RA/QA is responsible to the President for the overall administration of this Total Quality Program and for assuring that annual management reviews and resultant actions shall be documented and provided to all appropriate levels of management."

Company C

"To consistently provide products and services which meet or exceed the quality requirements of our customers through continuous improvement."

820.20(b) ORGANIZATION

The Requirement

820.20(b) Organization. Each manufacturer shall establish and maintain an adequate organizational structure to ensure that devices are designed and produced in accordance with the requirements of this part.

(1) Responsibility and authority. Each manufacturer shall establish the appropriate responsibility, authority, and interrelation of all personnel who manage, perform, and assess work affecting quality, and provide the independence and authority necessary to perform these tasks.

(2) Resources. Each manufacturer shall provide adequate resources, including the assignment of trained personnel, for management, performance of work, and assessment activities, including internal quality audits, to meet the requirements of this part.

(3) Management representative. Management with executive responsibility shall appoint, and document such appointment of, a member of management who, irrespective of other responsibilities, shall have established authority over and responsibility for:

(i) Ensuring that quality system requirements are effectively established and effectively maintained in accordance with this part; and

(ii) Reporting on the performance of the quality system to management with executive responsibility for review.

Discussion of the Requirement

It is a manufacturer's responsibility to create an organizational structure adequate to ensure that devices are produced in accordance with the manufacturer's quality system and with the GMP requirements. The FDA has clearly indicated that an adequate organizational structure is necessary not only to ensure compliance, but also to ensure a manufacturer's ability to consistently produce safe and effective devices. The type of organizational structure established will be determined by the volume and type of device(s) produced, the manufacturer's organizational goals, and the expectations and needs of customers.

Section 820.20(b) of the regulation requires each manufacturer to ensure that responsibility, authority, and organizational independence is provided to personnel who manage, perform, and verify work affecting quality. Section 820.20(b)(2) requires each manufacturer to provide adequate resources for the quality system. These resources include monetary as well as personnel resources.

Management with executive responsibility is required to appoint a member of management who has established authority and responsibility for ensuring that the quality system requirements are defined, documented, implemented, and maintained in accordance with GMP requirements. The management representative must have the independence to ensure that the quality system is not compromised, and the management representative is responsible for reporting to management with executive responsibility on the performance of the quality system.

Industry Practice

A specific organizational structure for executing a quality assurance program is not prescribed by the Quality System regulation. Past practices dictated that, where possible, a designated individual not having direct responsibility for the performance of a manufacturing operation be responsible for the QA program. However, FDA and industry are more concerned with the adequacy and appropriateness of QA activities than with organizational structure. With downsizing and streamlining, it is not always possible, practical, or efficient to have a separate QA function.

When a separate QA organization is in place, a manufacturer should not operate on the basis that this function has primary and direct responsibility for the quality of the product. To do so means that quality problems will not be solved in a timely manner because attention is directed toward the wrong organization. Rather, the QA organization is responsible for ensuring that attention is directed toward the correct department(s) if a quality problem arises.

Manufacturers design their quality systems to fit their specific needs. Many manufacturers have developed their own quality practices to be used on a day-to-day basis. Many have also become ISO 9001 or 9002 certified, and their quality practices are codified in the quality policy and quality manual. The quality policy and quality manual are developed to assist manufacturers in carrying out their daily quality responsibilities.

The quality system is a set of checks and double-checks on the product from design through distribution. Through company organization, structure, and compliance with ISO quality standards and the Quality System regulation, manufacturers have developed controls to ensure that their devices are produced to be safe and effective. Management provides resources for the quality system by establishing written procedures, personnel, and funds directed toward the quality effort.

Manufacturers that have appointed a management representative often designate a member of the quality function management team. The documenting of this appointment does not need to be elaborate; it is often noted on an organizational chart or referenced in the quality manual.

820.20(c) MANAGEMENT REVIEW

The Requirement

820.20(c) Management review. Management with executive responsibility shall review the suitability and effectiveness of the quality system at defined internals and with sufficient frequency according to established procedures to ensure that the quality system satisfies the requirements of this part and the manufacturer's established quality policy and objectives. The dates and results of quality system reviews shall be documented.

Discussion of the Requirement

The aim of the management review is for management with executive responsibility to conduct a broad review of the organization as a whole to determine if its quality policy is implemented and the quality objectives are being met. The review is also intended to ensure the continued adequacy and effectiveness of the quality system. All parts of the quality system are to be reviewed, but different areas may be reviewed at different times. The frequency of reviews should be defined and linked to the quality policy and objectives. A documented system that defines how management intends to review the quality system is required. The FDA has clearly indicated that written procedures are necessary to ensure the consistency and completeness of required reviews.

Although the regulation requires documentation of the management review results, FDA has decided not to request to inspect and copy the reports during routine inspections. This decision was intended to help ensure that the reviews are complete, candid, and of maximum use to the manufacturer. The FDA may require management with executive responsibility to certify in writing that the requirements of section 820.20(c) have been met. In addition, the written procedure for management review will be subject to inspection and copying.

Industry Practice

Many U.S. companies are ISO certified or in the process of obtaining ISO certification and already have a management review process and procedure in place. Gathering and presenting the information for management review is a responsibility often assigned to the quality assurance and/or regulatory affairs groups, who have day-to-day experience with quality systems and quality data.

The management review may include an evaluation of the organizational structure; the adequacy of staffing and resources; the achieved quality of the finished device relative to the quality objectives; and other information, including customer feedback (e.g., complaints, recalls), process and product performance, servicing information, audit results (internal, third-party, supplier), and any corrective or preventive actions taken.

It is up to a manufacturer to determine what constitutes a "sufficient frequency" for management reviews. Management should review the appropriateness of the review frequency, based on the findings of previous reviews. For established and compliant firms, an annual review may be sufficient. If there are known problems or if the quality system is not yet proven, "sufficient frequency" may mean fairly frequent.

A typical management review practice in industry is to convene a gathering of executive management. For ease of review, information may be presented in tabular or graphic form. Comparisons may be drawn with similar data in previous years to show improvement (or lack of improvement) relative to quality indicators. During the management review, representatives discuss the information they have obtained and determine whether additional resources, programs, or systems are appropriate to address any quality concerns. Both the review and the recommendations may be documented in minutes of the meeting.

In addition to meeting the ISO requirement for documented management review of quality systems, the vast majority of organizations hold periodic management meetings in which, among other issues, quality indicators are reviewed and discussed. Although not a part of the formal management review, these types of meetings are quite valuable in providing timely information and feedback to executive management regarding quality issues and quality progress.

The formal management review may also take the form of a written report on the quality system, which is circulated among top-level management. The written report, which may be prepared and reviewed as necessary, includes the same type of information on important quality indicators as is presented at a management review meeting. Written sign-offs, indicating that the report has been reviewed and understood, may be required as a means of documentation. Individual comments on the contents of the report may also be requested. This type of management review may be more efficient in terms of time, particularly in a large corporation, but lacks the opportunity for discussion and exchange of ideas that a meeting presents.

The effectiveness of management review as a tool for quality review and improvement depends, of course, on the commitment of top-level management to quality systems and products. This is a concept that FDA understands well and sees in practice often. Even though FDA will not routinely ask for information from management reviews, just as audit reports are not routinely requested, the effectiveness and adequacy of management review can be judged by reviewing other required quality records, including inspection and testing results for incoming, in-process, and finished devices, complaint files, and service reports. For this reason, a critical part of management review is to assess the information that FDA will see in terms of the quality policy and objectives and to ensure that appropriate preventive and corrective actions are underway when problems occur.

820.20(d) QUALITY PLANNING

The Requirement

820.20(d) Quality planning. Each manufacturer shall establish a quality plan which defines the quality practices, resources, and activities relevant to devices that are designed and manufactured. The manufacturer shall establish how the requirements for quality will be met.

Discussion of the Requirement

This section of the regulation requires manufacturers to define and document the procedures and instructions used to establish and implement the quality system. The quality system documentation must define the objectives and requirements for quality, including such elements as fitness for use, performance, safety, and reliability. A quality plan may be an independent document defining how the quality requirements will be met, or it may simply reference other procedures that make up the manufacturer's quality system.

Industry Practice

A quality plan shows how the quality system requirements are applied to a device or device type to ensure that it meets specifications and quality requirements. The purpose of a quality plan is to communicate the requirements and controls necessary to manufacture, test, and release product that meets customer needs. The quality plan covers all quality practices, resources, and activities at all stages of manufacturing, including design, procurement, production, and, when applicable, installation and service.

Many manufacturers do not currently have documents clearly identified as "quality plans." The FDA has not mandated a specific format for such plans. If a manufacturer chooses to create separate quality plans, those documents should be consistent, and appropriate cross-referenced, with other documents relating to the device. If the individual documents are appropriately and adequately structured, it is possible to achieve the application of the quality system elements or establishment of the quality plan through the DMR. If the DMR is used, the manufacturer's quality manual or other top-level procedure typically defines how, and which elements of, the DMR meet the requirements of section 820.20(d).

820.20(e) QUALITY SYSTEM PROCEDURES

The Requirement

> *820.20(e) Quality system procedures. Each manufacturer shall establish quality system procedures and instructions. An outline of the structure of the documentation used in the quality system shall be established where appropriate.*

Discussion of the Requirement

Manufacturers are required to develop and maintain effective quality system procedures for compliance with each aspect of the Quality System regulation. The complexity and structure of these instructions depends on the manufacturer, its organization, and the device being produced. The quality system procedures must be designed to ensure the safety and effectiveness of the device. When appropriate and required to define the quality system, the documentation structure must be summarized (see section 820.186, "Quality system record").

Industry Practice

The existing quality systems of many manufacturers comply with the intent of section 820.20(e), with the possible exception of the required outline of the documentation structure. Those manufacturers whose quality systems meet the requirements of an ISO 9000 standard typically have documented systems that include an outline, most often in the form of a quality manual.

While not an absolute requirement of the regulation, a quality manual provides a concise description of the quality system and the policies and procedures that implement it. The importance of a quality manual depends on the size of the company and the complexity of its documentation structure. The requirements of this section of the regulation can be easily met by a small manufacturer through one tier of documentation; for larger manufacturers, multiple tiers of documentation, including a top-level quality manual, are appropriate for compliance with the GMP requirements and for effective operation of the quality system.

The quality manual shows how each quality system requirement is met. It is common for a quality manual to include the manufacturer's quality policy, a description of the organization, and a summary of the quality system procedures with appropriate cross-references to more detailed documentation. Quality system procedures encompass system-related procedures as well as device-specific procedures for processes that help to ensure that the quality objectives are met. The quality manual can be one document supported by several tiers of documents, with each tier becoming progressively more detailed; together, they define the quality system.

820.22 QUALITY AUDIT

The Requirement

820.22 Quality audit. Each manufacturer shall establish procedures for quality audits and conduct such audits to assure that the quality system is in compliance with the established quality system requirements and to determine the effectiveness of the quality system. Quality audits shall be conducted by individuals who do not have direct responsibility for the matters being audited. Corrective action(s), including a reaudit of deficient matters, shall be taken when necessary. A report of the results of each quality audit, and reaudit(s) where taken shall be made and such reports shall be reviewed by management having responsibility for the matters audited. The dates and results of quality audits and reaudits shall be documented.

Discussion of the Requirement

This section requires each manufacturer to conduct a periodic internal review of the quality system to verify compliance with the Quality System regulation. A manufacturer must review all procedures to ensure adequacy and compliance with the regulation and determine whether the procedures are being effectively implemented at all times. This review applies to all activities relating to the quality system and areas of the company in which the quality system is implemented.

Manufacturers are required to establish written procedures for conducting quality audits. The procedures should detail the specific requirements for conducting quality audits and explain key aspects of the quality audit system. System requirements should include identification of areas and elements to be audited; scheduling of audits; standards to be used to conduct audits; auditor and/or audit team requirements; and audit preparation, records, reporting, corrective action, and closure.

Qualified individuals must be designated to conduct the quality audits. The FDA expects auditors to be independent of the function or element being audited. Independence needs to be maintained so that the auditor is objective enough to identify deficiencies within the function or element being audited and to assess whether corrective actions, if required, are adequate and have been implemented. The failure to have an independent auditor could result in an ineffective audit.

It is up to the manufacturer to decide when and how often audits should be conducted. The decision should be based on the performance of the quality-system activity, the difficulty of the activity, and prior history. It is expected that audits will be conducted at least annually. Regardless, the frequency of audits should be planned and such plans should be documented. Audits are required to cover all of a manufacturer's operations and all applicable elements of the regulation. Audits may be conducted at one time or in stages.

The results of quality audits, whether or not deficiencies are observed, are required to be documented. The FDA expects that audit results will be reviewed by management as part of the management review activities specified in section 820.20(c). Management is expected to identify and provide the resources needed to implement and follow up on corrective actions so that the recurrence of problems observed can be prevented and the safety, reliability, and effectiveness of the product ensured.

It is also expected by FDA that audit results will be provided to the individuals responsible for the operations audited and that these individuals will respond, when necessary, with a corrective action plan. When corrective action is identified, it is expected that such action will be taken in a timely manner and that a reaudit will be conducted to verify that the action has been taken and is effective. Such verification should be documented.

As indicated in section 820.180(c), it is FDA policy not to review audit results and audit reports. However, manufacturers are required to maintain records documenting audits and reaudits to demonstrate that audits have been completed as planned.

Industry Practice

The FDA's Compliance Program Guidance 7382.830, *Inspection of Medical Device Manufacturers*, instructs investigators to review audit procedures, the content of which should include at least the following elements: objectives, assignment of responsibilities, audit scope, evaluation criteria, and audit scheduling.

Audits address compliance with company policy, procedures, and specifications, as well as compliance with the Quality System regulation and the effectiveness of the manufacturer's quality system. Audit programs within industry vary from facility to facility, based in part on the resources available to conduct a successful audit.

Some device manufacturers do the minimum; they audit the entire quality system only once a year. Other manufacturers have implemented comprehensive audit schedules on a more frequent basis.

While there are numerous ways to design and implement an effective audit program, many manufacturers have found the following items to be useful elements of a documented audit procedure:

Scope: The scope defines which facilities and which functions or activities are affected by the procedure.

Audit Plan and Schedule: This part of the procedure describes how the plan and schedule are determined and approved and specifies the frequency of the audit. When determining the audit frequency, the manufacturer should consider the amount and seriousness of past audit observations. If no previous audits have been conducted, the manufacturer should identify, based on management review activities, potential problem areas or areas of major quality impact and focus on those areas first.

Responsibilities: This part of the procedure defines responsibilities for executing the audit system, developing the audit plan, assigning auditors, developing and implementing corrective action plans, reporting findings, and reviewing findings by management.

Auditor Requirements: This part of the procedure defines the required training, experience, independence, and composition of the audit team (where teams are used) and addresses the use of consultants. Independence is crucial to the effectiveness of a successful audit program. To maintain auditor independence, auditors should not audit any areas or functions for which they have functional responsibility.

Auditors should have management support to conduct audits and report observations objectively. This is usually accomplished by having the auditor report directly to the management representative responsible for the quality program. Another option is to assign the auditor direct or dotted-line responsibility to the president or CEO, or even to have the auditor report directly to the president or CEO.

Auditors can be quality assurance personnel, personnel from other areas within the company, or consultants. Some small companies use consultants to address the concern about independence. Larger manufacturers sometimes use consultants to obtain an outside verification of adequacy of compliance. Audits are usually conducted by one auditor, but some companies, particularly those that are seeking or have obtained ISO certification/CE marking, have gone to an audit team approach of two or more auditors.

Audit Standards: Guidance is provided on the standards to be used by auditors in conducting audits (e.g., the Quality System regulation, ISO 13485, company policies and procedures, the device master record).

Audit Process: The details of the audit process are described (e.g., interviewing, observing, tracing, taking notes, using checklists, reporting audit findings, debriefing on a daily or other specified basis, opening and closing meetings). The procedure should identify any checklists to be used and how these checklists are to be approved. Checklists are a series of questions that review the function being audited to determine the effectiveness and compliance of that function. A checklist acts as a guide to the auditors to ensure that all aspects of the quality system are assessed. Notes and observations indicating compliance or noncompliance are recorded on the checklist. Some manufacturers rate observations as major or minor based upon the risk associated with the noncompliance raised.

Results and Reports: This part of the procedure describes the method of recording audit findings (forms, checklists, reports), preparing the final report, and issuing the report to responsible parties, including management. The procedure should identify the time frames that responsible individuals have to provide a response and implement corrective actions. Audit reports should be part of management review activities. Any assistance required by executive management to effect corrective action should be documented.

Systems for documenting and formally reporting audit findings vary from company to company and may take the form of audit checklists, audit records, or audit reports. In almost all instances, a summary cover letter will be generated with the observations attached or included as part of the formal audit report. For FDA review purposes, manufacturers typically maintain records to demonstrate compliance with the audit requirements of the Quality System regulation. These records typically take the form of an audit log or a certification letter. Such records would include the audit date(s), the name(s) of the auditor(s) who conducted the audit, the scope of the audit, and the date the audit was closed. Audit records are typically maintained by the audit system manager or the quality assurance function.

Corrective Action: This part of the procedure describes the steps for requesting, implementing, and verifying by reaudits the corrective action, and it addresses responsibilities and timeliness. Corrective action should encompass

- a) identification of the root cause of the problem;
- b) the action to correct the specific problem;
- c) the action to correct the root cause;
- d) identification of other areas and/or products affected by the problem; and,
- e) the action to correct any problems with other areas and/or products.

As a practical matter, almost all audit observations require corrective action. It is the level of corrective action that varies according to circumstances. When an observation is made, corrective action is requested from the management representative of the audited area within a reasonable time. An investigation into the cause of the noncompliance is conducted before corrective action is defined and initiated. At the time corrective action is implemented, or shortly afterwards, the auditor returns to the area to verify that corrective action has been taken and is effective. In rare instances, implementation of corrective action may be verified by review of documentation.

Follow-Up: This part of the procedure should address how follow-up audits are to be conducted and documented. During follow-up audits, it is necessary to evaluate and verify the implementation and effectiveness of corrective actions taken to remedy audit observations.

Audit Closure: This part of the procedure describes the methods of determining that the audit loop has been completed (e.g., verification of corrective actions, completion of any logs, certification and maintenance of audit files).

820.25 PERSONNEL

The Requirement

820.25 Personnel

(a) General. Each manufacturer shall have sufficient personnel with the necessary education, background, training, and experience to assure that all activities required by this part are correctly performed.

(b) Training. Each manufacturer shall establish procedures for identifying training needs and ensure that all personnel are trained to adequately perform their assigned responsibilities. Training shall be documented.

(1) As part of their training, personnel shall be made aware of device defects which may occur from the improper performance of their specific jobs.

(2) Personnel who perform verification and validation activities shall be made aware of defects and errors that may be encountered as part of their job functions.

Discussion of the Requirement

This section requires each manufacturer to employ sufficient personnel, as determined by the requirements of the company's quality system, to establish procedures to identify training needs, to provide appropriate training for personnel, and to maintain records of training.

It is up to the manufacturer to determine what constitutes "sufficient" personnel with the necessary qualifications to perform their functions. The manufacturer must ensure that personnel assigned to particular functions are properly equipped and that they have the necessary education, background, training, and experience to perform the function correctly and ensure that devices are produced according to specifications.

A manufacturer must have an established procedure that includes the identification of training needs. The training program must ensure that each employee understands both the job function itself and the GMP requirements pertaining to that particuluar job function, including how the job relates to the overall quality system. In addition, employee training is required to cover the consequences of improper performance so that employees are aware of defects that they should look for and of the effect their actions can have on the safety and effectiveness of the device.

For the quality system to function as planned, all personnel are required to be properly trained. Each function, not only those affecting quality, must be viewed as integral to all other functions. All personnel must be trained in the functions and procedures that they will encounter while performing their assigned jobs.

Industry Practice

No matter how effective quality and production systems are as concepts, people still play the major role in producing a quality product. Training is more than an administrative function; it should be continuous and appropriate for each employee's job function.

The first step in meeting the requirements of section 820.25 is to select and hire appropriate employees. There are no documented guidelines from FDA concerning the exact education, background, and experience needed to satisfy the intent of the regulation. In Compliance Program 7382.830, *Inspection of Medical Device Manufacturers,* FDA instructs investigators to look for situations in which personnel failed to perform a job or performed it inadequately due to insufficient training. By extension, FDA investigators may look for instances in which inadequate personnel education, background, or experience adversely affected device safety and efficacy.

Although prior GMP experience is preferred for certain positions, it is not mandated by the regulation. Personnel should, however, have the necessary education and skills to perform the tasks required of the position. Upper and middle levels of management are often exempt from job-specific training requirements. These individuals usually possess the required education and/or experience when hired. They are subject to general training programs (e.g., GMP requirements, ISO, orientation) that are considered company-wide. If an individual is hired who does not possess the required background for a given position, as noted in the job description for that position, it is the company's responsibility to make sure that training is provided and documented in a reasonable time period.

A manufacturer's written training program typically addresses

    a) responsibility for training programs;
    b) methods of identifying training needs and qualifications of personnel;
    c) identification of those jobs that require formal training and GMP requirements training;
    d) methods of documenting job descriptions;
    e) methods of determining success of training (e.g., testing, documented follow-up);
    f) methods of documenting activities and maintaining the documentation; and,
    g) retraining requirements.

General GMP training is routinely provided to all employees by device manufacturers. Such training is provided at the time the employee is hired and then annually, or as needed, thereafter. In addition, depending on the job skills required, specialized training may be provided for specific job functions. The degree of training required, including GMP training, will depend on the employee and on the complexity of the position. These requirements should be established and documented.

Lack of training, as reflected in instances of negligence, poor operating techniques, or the inability of employees to perform their functions properly, can lead to defective products and, sometimes, to regulatory or liability issues. Management should be diligent in looking for factors that indicate a need for employee training. Evidence of personnel problems or training problems might include an excessive number of in-process rejects and failures, employees' lack of knowledge of documentation, or an excessive number of complaints.

Identifying Training Needs. Job titles may be used to identify the general training areas required. Specific training requirements may be listed by department, facility work area, and then by job function. For example, training on GMP requirements as well as a general facility and production overview would be required for all job titles. Departmental breakdown would identify the specific training required for personnel working in the manufacturing department versus the QA department. More specialized training may be required in particular work areas; for example, training in aseptic practices or specific safety precautions might be needed. Job function training would include task-specific instructions, such as how to use a particulate analyzer or a pH meter. All such requirements should be documented in a formal, approved procedure, which includes the format of the training program.

Developing Training Systems/Manuals. Consistent, documented programs are developed so that consideration is given to all potential training requirements for the personnel in the applicable areas. This approach is especially helpful if there is no department specifically responsible for training and training is implemented by various people, such as departmental supervisors. A consistent list of requirements is established for each job function, and the applicability is determined. For example, a training program checklist might include the following elements:

a) general GMP requirements training;
b) specific GMP requirements training;
c) documentation requirements;
d) standard operating procedures;
e) equipment considerations;
f) personnel safety/first aid;
g) applicable techniques for ensuring product safety and efficacy;
h) security;
i) hazardous materials;
j) specific skills required (current and updates as needed);
k) hygiene;
l) required certifications (current and updates as needed);
m) literature references;
n) task practice exercises; and,
o) potential defects and ramifications.

When the applicable areas of the checklist have been determined for each job function, a training manual is developed to include the requirements.

Training programs must cover contract and temporary employees. The extent of training versus supervision depends primarily on the length of time the employee will be working and the job function that the employee is performing. All contract and temporary employees should receive basic GMP and company orientation training. The company procedure should define a contract employee versus a temporary employee. Because contract employees are often long-term, they may require the same level of training as permanent employees. Constant, direct supervision and basic task-related instructions should suffice for temporary employees.

Implementing Training. Training is implemented as outlined in the facility training program. A schedule is developed to allow for personnel replacement, if necessary, for budget considerations, and for scheduling of outside training resources, if required.

Maintaining Records. Various methods are utilized to maintain employee training records. Depending on the database used (electronic or manual), records may be maintained by cross-referencing to a specific procedure, task, facility area, training session, or other category. Records may also be referenced to each employee or department.

In large companies, maintenance of training records may be a joint responsibility of the human resources (HR) and operating departments. For instance, educational accomplishments, external training, prior training, job descriptions, orientation records, and general ongoing training (e.g., basic GMP requirements) may be maintained by the HR department. Records of internal job responsibilities, ongoing job-related training, and specific task-related training may be maintained by the operating department supervisor/manager. In smaller firms, one department typically maintains all training records.

A manufacturer's requirements for training documentation usually include the employee's name and signature; the date of hire; the document/program trained against; the name and signature of the person by whom the employee was trained; the date of training; and, the type of training (e.g., GMP, orientation, incoming inspection).

Training Updates. The Quality System regulation requires that manufacturers make certain that all personnel are adequately trained. Therefore, training should be updated as needed. To meet part of this requirement, many manufacturers provide periodic retraining in basic GMP requirements and the application of the regulation. "Periodic" typically translates to annual retraining. Retraining requirements should be specified in the company's training procedure.

While there is no specific GMP requirement for retraining when a new procedure is written or when an existing procedure has been changed or updated, many manufacturers retrain the affected personnel or make a notation in the change order explaining why retraining is not necessary. There are other methods of acceptable training (e.g., baseline and job skills training) that would not require retraining on a revision-by-revision basis. Retraining may be required under special circumstances, as when, for example, numerous customer complaints have been received, procedures are being performed improperly, or an excessive number of product defects are occurring.

DESIGN

CHAPTER 8. DESIGN CONTROLS (SUBPART C)

820.30 DESIGN CONTROLS

820.30(a) GENERAL

The Requirement

820.30(a) General. (1) Each manufacturer of any class III or class II device, and the class I devices listed in paragraph (a)(2) of this section, shall establish and maintain procedures to control the design of the device in order to ensure that specified design requirements are met.

(2) The following class I devices are subject to design controls:

(i) Devices automated with computer software; and

(ii) The devices listed in the chart below.

Section	Device
868.6810	Catheter, Tracheobronchial Suction
878.4460	Glove, Surgeon's
880.6760	Restraint, Protective
892.5650	System, Applicator, Radionuclide, Manual
892.5740	Source, Radionuclide Teletherapy

Discussion of the Requirement

The FDA has identified improvements in safety and effectiveness as the objective of the application of design controls. Design control is the process of controlling and monitoring the design of a device to ensure that specified design requirements are met. The design control requirements of the Quality System regulation are applicable to all class II and class III devices. The design control requirements also apply to selected class I devices, outlined above, and to class I devices automated with computer software. Software accessories to class I devices also must be developed according to design controls even though the parent class I device may be exempt.

Design control requirements are not intended to apply during the research phase (i.e., to the development of concepts or to feasibility studies). After it is decided that a design will be developed, a plan must be generated for establishing the adequacy of the design requirements and ensuring that the design that will eventually be released to production meets the approved requirements. Design controls are applicable to investigational device exemption (IDE) devices.

The FDA does not intend the design control requirements to be retroactive, and section 820.30 does not require manufacturers to apply such requirements to already distributed devices. However, the design control requirements do apply to changes affecting already distributed devices.

Industry Practice

It has been widely recognized that production controls and process validation are not enough to produce high-quality medical devices. The concept of quality has evolved from quality control (inspect and test) to quality assurance (process validation, "build in quality") to the quality system, in which quality is designed into the device and the focus is on the customer. Industry is supportive of the harmonization of the GMP requirements with the ISO 9001 quality system standard, which encompasses design control.

Unsafe and ineffective devices are often the result of informal development that does not ensure the proper establishment of design requirements and does not provide for proper assessment of the device requirements, which are necessary to develop a medical device with the proper level of safety and effectiveness for the intended use of the device and the needs of the user.

As the sophistication of devices increases, the benefits associated with the application of design controls become more apparent. Successful manufacturers have implemented design control techniques for new products because they have experienced shortened, more predictable development schedules and reduced R&D costs as a result of establishing better requirements and identifying problems or errors early in the design process.

820.30(b) DESIGN AND DEVELOPMENT PLANNING

The Requirement

> *820.30(b) Design and development planning. Each manufacturer shall establish and maintain plans that describe or reference the design and development activities and define responsibility for implementation. The plans shall identify and describe the interfaces with different groups or activities that provide, or result in, input to the design and development process. The plans shall be reviewed, updated, and approved as design and development evolves.*

Discussion of the Requirement

This section of the Quality System regulation clearly delineates the need for application of design controls in a prospective manner; that is, the design must be addressed in a plan prepared prior to the formal development process. The design and development plan may exist across multiple documents; for example, there may be separate plans for hardware and software. The plan should describe the development process that the manufacturer intends to follow, and it should be specific to the organization and to the complexity of the product. The plan should include or reference any relevant standard operating procedures (SOPs), thereby addressing the following elements of the design and development process:

a) key tasks and minimum design reviews for each phase;
b) development practices;

c) quality practices and verification methodology, when known;

d) coding guidelines for software;

e) record-keeping and documentation;

f) resources (e.g., people, tools, facilities);

g) risk analysis methods; and,

h) schedule.

When the design control requirements become effective, they will apply to designs that are within the design and development phase at that time. For each such device, the manufacturer will be expected to have established a design and development plan, to have identified the design stage of the device, and to comply with the established design and development plan and the applicable parts of section 820.30 from that point forward to completion. However, it will not be mandatory for designs to be recycled through previous phases that have been completed.

The FDA requires manufacturers to establish the appropriate responsibility for activities affecting quality and emphasizes that the assignment of specific responsibilities is important to the success of the design control program and to achieving compliance with the regulation.

In any design process, additional information on system capabilities and evolving customer requirements will mandate changes. If the process changes from the originally planned approach, the design and development plan must be updated to reflect those changes, especially when activities related to the verification and validation of the device are affected. The FDA recognizes that changes to the plan may be necessary and expects such changes to be implemented in a formal manner (i.e., reviewed and approved).

Industry Practice

Historically, many manufacturers did not develop new products according to a formal design and development plan. However, critical schedule demands and time-to-market objectives have increased awareness of the benefits of formal planning. Today, the manufacturers that are most successful in new development invest time up front to plan the activities and resources required to build quality into new developmental products. Increasing product complexity and evolving customer expectations have dictated the need for more sophisticated development practices based on formal, upfront planning.

Design and development plans vary from simple to complex, depending on the technologies that are incorporated into the device under development. Key development tasks to be included in the plan may relate to hardware, electronics, software, sterility, and biocompatibility of materials. Development milestones trigger the performance of design reviews, which are specified in the design and development plan.

Manufacturers are often plagued by inadequate communication between engineering, R&D, and other departments. This problem can be reduced to a great extent by describing in the design and development plan the responsibilities of all affected departments (e.g., engineering, R&D, manufacturing, marketing, QA, regulatory affairs, and service), including the information that is received and transmitted.

Schedules may be developed and maintained by manufacturers with the help of tools such as program evaluation review technique (PERT) and Gantt charts. These tools and techniques aid in project planning, evaluating the effect of deviations on development schedules, determining the probability of meeting deadlines, and identifying bottlenecks. For simpler projects, spreadsheets and flow charts are often found to be more useful.

820.30(c) DESIGN INPUT

The Requirement

820.30(c) Design input. Each manufacturer shall establish and maintain procedures to ensure that the design requirements relating to a device are appropriate and address the intended use of the device, including the needs of the user and patient. The procedures shall include a mechanism for addressing incomplete, ambiguous, or conflicting requirements. The design input requirements shall be documented and shall be reviewed and approved by a designated individual(s). The approval, including the date and signature of the individual(s) approving the requirements, shall be documented.

Discussion of the Requirement

Section 820.3(f) defines design input as "the physical and performance requirements of a device that are used as a basis for device design."

The design input defines product performance, safety, and reliability characteristics, environmental limits, physical attributes, compatibility with other devices, applicable standards, regulatory requirements, packaging specifications, and labeling. The intended use of the device must address the needs of users and patients, and it must be explicit in the label claims.

The design input must be captured in a set of requirements that are translated into a formal specification(s) that is reviewed and approved by the project team and placed under formal change control. When changes are made to the design input, the changes to requirements must be formally reviewed and evaluated, and the specification(s) revised to reflect the changes. All affected parties must be notified to assure that any potential adverse consequences are considered.

The FDA recognizes the design input as the basis of the design validation program. Failure to have an accurate and complete design input results in failure to demonstrate design validation. Simply providing a large number of test procedures and results that cannot be mapped to requirements does not constitute adequate evidence of validation. Thus, the design input should be testable, completely define the system functions to be implemented, be consistent in terminology and specifications, and be understandable by the target audience. That audience includes the marketing department, which represents user expectations; the engineering/R&D department, which is responsible for implementation; and the QA department, which is responsible for assuring that target quality goals are met.

Section 820.30(c) requires the manufacturer to ensure that the design input requirements are appropriate (i.e., that the device will perform its intended use and meet the needs of the user). In doing so, the manufacturer must assess and set the proper level of safety and effectiveness commensurate with the intended use of the device.

Industry Practice

The design input phase is also known as the requirements phase in the traditional engineering development model.

Successful design and development manufacturers realize that using marketing specifications alone as the basis for design is not acceptable. A testable formal specification that completely defines the system is necessary to ensure product completeness and acceptance. Failure to define requirements results in the inability to effectively determine the completeness and adequacy of the development program.

Industry often uses the team approach to perform design reviews. Designs are reviewed and evaluated by all disciplines necessary to ensure that the design input requirements are appropriate and adequately address the intended use of the device and user/patient needs.

One of the tools used by manufacturers to translate the design input into specifications is "Quality Function Deployment," the systematic determination of the design specifications that best satisfy users' needs and the intended use of the device. The design input is worked by a cross-functional team to translate customer requirements into design specifications. This activity is usually lead by the R&D project manager. Other tools used by industry are brainstorming, pareto charts, and affinity diagrams to categorize the design input and reach agreement on the performance and safety specifications of the device.

Relevant information for design input may come from customer complaints, sales and service data, focus groups, customer surveys, R&D, and/or marketing. Customer complaints, including MDRs, form a quality feedback loop for distributed products that drives continuous quality improvements. Quality assurance trend analyses can help define performance and safety requirements for both product improvements and new product development. Data from service reports help determine reliability and the possible need for design changes. Marketing is often the voice of the customer, and marketing tools include focus groups and customer surveys.

820.30(d) DESIGN OUTPUT

The Requirement

820.30(d) Design output. Each manufacturer shall establish and maintain procedures for defining and documenting design output in terms that allow an adequate evaluation of conformance to design input requirements. Design output procedures shall contain or make reference to acceptance criteria and shall ensure that those design outputs that are essential for the proper functioning of the device are identified. Design output shall be documented, reviewed, and approved before release. The approval, including the date and signature of the individual(s) approving the output, shall be documented.

Discussion of the Requirement

Design output is defined in section 820.3(g) as "the results of a design effort at each design phase and at the end of the total design effort. The finished design output is the basis for the device master record. The total finished device output consists of the device, its packaging and labeling, and the device master record." This section of the Quality System regulation requires a manufacturer to define and document design output and to ensure that the output meets the approved design input requirements.

Design output occurs throughout the design process; therefore, this GMP requirement is applicable to all phases of design. The total finished design output includes the device, device and component specifications, packaging, labeling, production specifications and drawings, and quality assurance specifications and procedures. Design output documents serve as the foundation for the DMR. In accordance with quality record-keeping practices, all design outputs must be reviewed and approved prior to release.

Industry Practice

Design output is not just a design phase, but rather the documentation of all activities performed during the design process to verify correct implementation of design input requirements and to support final design specifications. Design output culminates with the completion of the final design documentation and the formal release of the DMR.

Examples of design output generated during the design process include drawings, schematics, test procedures, laboratory notebooks, hardware configuration specifications, software specifications, design review records, risk analysis data, technical reports, component qualifications, performance test plans and reports, and validation and verification plans and reports. In addition to the product of the design process, final design output includes labeling, specifications (device, subassembly, component, software, packaging), production procedures, installation and service procedures (if applicable), and quality procedures and criteria. These are the elements that make up the product's DMR.

The level of documentation provided as design output varies based on device complexity and size. For large systems, multiple layers of design documentation, defining separate subsystem specifications and design descriptions, may be appropriate. Manufacturers have learned that design documentation is essential to capture the investment spent on the development of new product systems. Until a design is documented, it belongs to the author (programmer or designer), not to the company. If a design is not documented, the knowledge base leaves as soon as the author leaves the company. The cost of changes and maintenance is increased substantially for product systems that fail to have adequate design documentation.

820.30(e) DESIGN REVIEW

The Requirement

820.30(e) Design review. Each manufacturer shall establish and maintain procedures to ensure that formal documented reviews of the design results are planned and conducted at appropriate stages of the device's design development. The procedures shall ensure that participants at each design review include representatives of all functions concerned with the design stage being reviewed and an individual(s) who does not have direct responsibility for the design stage being reviewed, as well as any specialists needed. The results of a design review, including identification of the design, the date, and the individual(s) performing the review, shall be documented in the design history file (the DHF).

Discussion of the Requirement

The purpose of conducting design reviews during the design process is to ensure that the design satisfies the design input requirements for the intended use of the device and the needs of the user. Design review includes the review of design verification activities to determine whether the design output meets the functional and operational requirements; that the design is compatible with components and other accessories; that safety, reliability, service, and maintenance requirements are met; and that labeling and other regulatory requirements are satisfied. Section 820.3(h) defines design review as "a documented, comprehensive, systematic examination of a design to evaluate the adequacy of the design requirements, to evaluate the capability of the design to meet these requirements, and to identify problems." Early phases of the design process or design output cannot be subjected to test but are best evaluated through review techniques. The essence of design controls is the formal review of the specifications to support the detection and remedy of errors as early as possible in the design process.

Formal reviews are to be conducted at "appropriate stages" (e.g., major decision points) of the design process. The manufacturer has the ultimate responsibility for defining when reviews are to be conducted and the number of reviews to be conducted. The number of reviews should be based on the size and complexity of the design.

All review activities should be documented with a list of the participants, a description of the topics or issues discussed, and the checklists used for evaluation (as applicable). Documentation, including meeting minutes from design reviews, agendas for proposed design review meetings, action item lists, and follow-up reports, is to be included in the DHF to support evidence of reviews.

An independent party who is not directly responsible for the design is required to participate in design reviews. The level of independence required for the reviewer is up to the manufacturer. In all cases, the reviewer should have adequate expertise to perform the review effectively. The review activities performed should focus on the identification of errors (i.e, failures to meet user or patient needs and intended uses).

Industry Practice

Industry-leading companies recognize the benefits of formal design reviews and frequently provide training to personnel on effective review techniques. In addition, the most successful manufacturers track review effectiveness and use the errors found in reviews as the basis for identifying process improvement activities. When errors are found during reviews, attempts are made to define changes to the design process that might lead to prevention of the errors in future development efforts.

Documents and other items essential to a design review meeting include a meeting agenda, all applicable specifications, drawings, manuals, test data, the results of special studies, mock-ups, breadboards, in-process hardware, finished hardware, and test methods. Review results and action items should be documented in meeting minutes.

Design reviews may include a system requirements review, a system design review, a software specification review, a preliminary design review, a critical design review, and a test readiness review. The usual participants include, as appropriate, manufacturing, quality assurance, regulatory, engineering, marketing, servicing, purchasing, R&D, preclinical, and clinical personnel.

The outcomes of design review meetings are typically documented and filed in the DHF. Identified action items are tracked to a conclusion, often by means of forms. Action items are frequently part of the agenda of the next review.

820.30(f) DESIGN VERIFICATION and 820.30(g) DESIGN VALIDATION

The Requirement

820.30 (f) Design verification. Each manufacturer shall establish and maintain procedures for verifying the device design. Design verification shall confirm that the design output meets the design input requirements. The results of the design verification, including identification of the design, method(s), the date, and the individual(s) performing the verification, shall be documented in the DHF.

820.30 (g) Design validation. *Each manufacturer shall establish and maintain procedures for validating the device design. Design validation shall be performed under defined operating conditions on initial production units, lots, or batches, or their equivalents. Design validation shall ensure that devices conform to defined user needs and intended uses and shall include testing of production units under actual or simulated use conditions. Design validation shall include software validation and risk analysis, where appropriate. The results of the design validation, including identification of the design, method(s), the date, and the individual(s) performing the validation, shall be documented in the DHF.*

Discussion of the Requirement

According to section 820.3(z), validation "means confirmation by examination and provision of objective evidence that the particular requirements for a specific intended use can be consistently fulfilled." In section 820.3(z)(2), design validation is defined as "establishing by objective evidence that device specifications conform with user needs and intended use(s)." Verification is defined in 820.3(aa) as "confirmation by examination and provision of objective evidence that specified requirements have been fulfilled."

Verification consists of specific activities performed during the design and development process that ensure that the defined process is being followed correctly and that the product specifications are met. Typical verification activities are documented inspections, tests, and objective evaluations.

Design validation follows successful design verification; design verification is not a substitute for design validation. Design validation should be performed under defined operating conditions and on multiple initial production lots or batches. Validation may also be carried out in earlier stages, prior to initial production. It may be necessary to perform multiple validations if there are different intended uses.

Production units must be included in the design validation and tested under conditions similar to those that are expected to be experienced in the user environment. This aspect of validation may require coordination with process validation activities, as defined in section 820.75 of the Quality System regulation. Tests in this phase of design control are simulated-use tests, use tests, or clinical studies, depending on the technology. Design validation includes product software validation and risk analysis.

It is inappropriate to assume that merely testing for satisfaction of requirements can provide adequate confidence in the correctness of a design. The testing must certainly address the defined requirements and also must target the actual environment or, where this may not be possible, an environment that simulates the actual use conditions. The validation tests also should address use by intended users, as the actual use of a device often does not directly coincide with that envisioned by the designers. Users may attempt to use a device in ways that were not anticipated during the development process. Stress testing by those unfamiliar with the design is a valuable technique of identifying potential error conditions.

The Quality System regulation requires the manufacturer to conduct a risk assessment that identifies potential safety risks, their severity, and the probability of their occurrence. The techniques that are most widely recognized for the performance of risk analyses are fault tree analysis (FTA) and failure modes and effects analysis (FMEA).

Software that is a part or component of, or an accessory to, a device must be validated. The FDA's *Reviewer Guidance for Computer Controlled Medical Devices Undergoing 510(k) Review*, issued in August 1991, describes software development methodologies, verification and validation activities, and risk analysis activities.*

The results of design validation and verification testing must be archived in the DHF.

Industry Practice

What is needed for verification and validation is determined by the product characteristics, predicate product knowledge, and the regulatory plan. For a product that will undergo premarket approval to demonstrate safety and effectiveness, more extensive testing will usually be necessary than for a product that will be cleared through a 510(k) premarket notification to establish equivalency to a product already on the market. Testing usually begins with working prototypes or breadboards and may be repeated as design changes are made. Typical verification tests include, where applicable

   a) comparative tests with a proven design;
   b) simulated use in the laboratory;
   c) animal model tests;
   d) biocompatibility tests;
   e) material/device compatibility tests;
   f) functional tests after sterilization;
   g) prototype tests;
   h) reliability tests;
   i) performance tests;
   j) tests of compatibility with other devices; and
   k) environmental tests.

For software, typical verification activities include code reviews, schematic reviews, unit and component tests, integration tests, and alternate calculation demonstrations.

There are many standards and guidelines that a manufacturer can research to identify expected tests. Product-specific guidance documents are available from FDA's Division of Small Manufacturers Assistance (DSMA) through "Facts On Demand." Other standards are available from the Ameri-

---

*A draft revision of this guidance document, entitled *ODE Guidance for the Content of Premarket Submissions for Medical Devices Containing Software,* was made available for comment on September 3, 1996.

can Society for Testing and Materials (ASTM), the American National Standards Institute (ANSI), the International Electrotechnical Commission (IEC), AAMI, and ISO.

The most common tool used in industry for risk analysis is FMEA, which is a systematic procedure by which potential design inadequacies that may adversely affect safety and performance can be identified and mitigated early in the development process. Potential risks are analyzed for normal-use, abuse, and misuse conditions. If any risk is judged unacceptable, it should be reduced to acceptable levels by appropriate means, such as redesign or warnings, among others. When conducted after changes are implemented, the FMEA technique also provides a means of verifying corrective actions. Assessing potential risk conditions associated with a device is no longer just an FDA regulatory requirement, but is now recognized as a key business strategy to prevent possible injury and to document due diligence in the design and development process.

Manufacturers have recognized the need to embrace formal verification and validation programs. It is understood that multiple levels of testing are essential to gain confidence in the correct functioning of complex devices. The primary responsibility for verification and validation is commonly placed on the R&D or engineering group. Quality assurance is typically assigned responsibility for audits, participation in reviews, safety risk assessment documentation, and independent testing.

One recognized practice for formally documenting the results of design validation activities is as follows:

a) Review and approve results.

b) Reflect the documentation of discrete test values or measurements in the results, where appropriate, and not merely a check mark to signify the completion of a test step.

c) Complete all required spaces on the test procedure forms or document as not applicable.

d) Address all deviations from defined test procedures in a test report addendum.

820.30(h) DESIGN TRANSFER

The Requirement

820.30(h) Design transfer. Each manufacturer shall establish and maintain procedures to ensure that the device design is correctly translated into production specifications.

Discussion of the Requirement

Except for validation of initial production units, design transfer is the final phase of product development and is the bridge between product design and product manufacturing. It is a transfer of knowledge in the form of documentation from product development to the manufacturing function. The released DMR is part of design output and is the basis for any additional documentation produced by other departments. Section 820.30(h) requires that a formal process be established to assure that the transfer of the design is effectively communicated to the manufacturing group.

The FDA has heightened attention to manufacturing processes and the adequacy of verification and validation. Tests performed on manufactured products should be related to key product safety and effectiveness requirements identified during development. See Chapter 16 for a detailed discussion of the GMP requirements for manufacturing process validation.

Proper testing of devices produced using the same methods and procedures as those to be used in routine production will help prevent distribution of unacceptable devices. While FDA has not mandated a specific number of lots or devices to be tested, the agency expects design validation to be carried out on initial production units, according to accepted statistical techniques.

The agency does not intend this section to prohibit manufacturers from beginning production until all design activities are completed. The intent of the requirement is to ensure that all design specifications released to production have been approved and verified or validated before they are implemented as part of the production process.

Industry Practice

For successful design transfer to occur, manufacturers find that communication between manufacturing and R&D needs to be initiated during the early development phases and continued throughout the product life cycle. In addition, whenever changes in the device design are proposed, the implications for manufacturing are considered.

Historically, the interface between R&D and manufacturing has not been very effective. Research and development groups have often simply "tossed" specifications over to manufacturing and failed to ensure that the specifications are well understood or effectively implemented. The results of this ad hoc process have been increased manufacturing costs, inefficient and redundant testing during manufacturing, and product field failures. The best practices today include coordination with manufacturing personnel early in the design process to ensure that design decisions take into consideration manufacturability and an overall test strategy that identifies component, subsystem, and final acceptance test procedures.

Industry practices include the following:

a) Manufacturing personnel participate in the design process up front to assure that appropriate built-in test functions are defined and adequate access is available to examine performance parameters.

b) Manufacturability is considered in design decisions, including cost of production equipment, impact on manufacturing processes, use of off-the-shelf components, and commonality of parts with existing and projected product lines.

c) A total test strategy is defined for the product. The test strategy, which may be derived from the design verification protocols, addresses test points appropriate to verify that the manufacturing operation has produced parts or product that meet specifications. The test strategy should encompass activities from component-level tests to final acceptance testing.

In the design transfer phase, preproduction specifications and documentation are transferred to manufacturing/production control. The transfer may not include the whole device; some parts may be released sooner than others. The team approach is more efficient and effective than a hand-off from R&D to manufacturing. Members of the design transfer team should include manufacturing engineering, document control, purchasing, quality assurance, and technical support. In order to have released documentation, validation and verification activities will have been completed.

Prior to the start of production, process control procedures, quality control procedures, sampling plans, testing/inspection instructions, maintenance/calibration/cleaning procedures, and training procedures are usually developed. Personnel training occurs before initial production and is continued thereafter as needed.

Freezing the device design is a difficult step, but it must be taken in consideration of development schedules, clinical trials, and regulatory submissions. A design review prior to and at completion of pilot production is recommended.

Although described as the last phase of design control, design transfer is not conducted sequentially only in the last phase of development. It begins early in the design control process, with manufacturing participating in the design team to assure a manufacturable design.

820.30(i) DESIGN CHANGES

The Requirement

820.30 (i) Design changes. Each manufacturer shall establish and maintain procedures for the identification, documentation, validation or where appropriate verification, review, and approval of design changes before their implementation.

Discussion of the Requirement

Manufacturers are required to have procedures to ensure that after design requirements are established and approved, changes to the design requirements are also reviewed, validated, and approved. Design output documentation consists of the final design specifications, which are often subject to changes during the development process. Changes to design specifications, once validated and accepted, must be subject to a formal change control process. Any changes to specifications must be subjected to the same level of controls and reviews as were applicable to the initial development effort. Such controls include review and approval by individuals in the same functions/organizations as those who signed off originally.

When changes are made, the validation tests that were developed for the initial release must be executed unless a rationale can be provided to support execution of only a limited subset of the test cases or no tests at all.

It is not the intent of the Quality System regulation to mandate that all design changes be documented and evaluated to the same extent, although they must all be documented and evaluated. The level of documentation and evaluation should be in direct proportion to the significance of the change.

Design changes that could potentially have significant effects on safety or performance must be reviewed to determine if a new 510(k) or a supplement to a PMAA will be required.

Industry Practice

Formal change control programs are essential to manage the complexity of most devices. Many manufacturers control revisions with an automated system to track which changes are implemented in which manufacturing lots. Manufacturing resource planning systems are very effective in tracking subsystem and component revisions for specific products. Automated software configuration management systems are also very effective in tracking what changes are introduced into which software program releases.

One change control process, properly structured, can deal with all types of changes efficiently (e.g., minor, major, or temporary changes).

Although most manufacturers evaluate all design changes, not all changes must be subjected to the same level of validation or verification. Some of the considerations involved in determining which changes should be selected for design control, and when, are as follows:

a) Key parameters of the initial design input need to be under control after they are approved. This is particularly true for complex designs.

b) The level of verification and validation to be performed for subcontractor changes is based on the complexity and safety implications of the proposed change as well as on the internal quality assurance activities of the subcontractor. In all cases, configuration management and control of changes is essential.

c) Change control may be needed for key parameters of a design undergoing clinical trials. Under current IDE policies, a significant change in the design may invalidate the clinical data.

d) After an element of a design is validated and accepted, later changes need to be controlled.

e) Design change control requirements apply to any change to a device, its labeling, or its packaging after it is released for production.

f) Manufacturing processes are also subject to change control.

820.30(j) DESIGN HISTORY FILE

The Requirement

820.30(j) Design history file. Each manufacturer shall establish and maintain a DHF for each type of device. The DHF shall contain or reference the records necessary to demonstrate that the design was developed in accordance with the approved design plan and the requirements of this part.

Discussion of the Requirement

Section 820.3(e) defines the design history file as "a compilation of records which describes the design history of a finished device." The DHF is intended to act as a repository for the data necessary to show compliance with the design plan and design control procedures by providing a complete design history of the finished device. The DHF must provide specific documentation showing the actions taken with regard to each device design. For a product family, the same DHF may be used for minor variations in a design, such as size differences.

Industry Practice

The level of formality with which companies maintain design documentation for new development efforts varies greatly. All successful manufacturers recognize the benefits of documenting the product design and design process: assurance that mistakes made in initial prototypes will not be repeated; the establishment of a baseline for evaluating quality throughout the design process and for designing the next generation of products; and evidence of compliance with procedures for liability and regulatory purposes.

One approach to organizing a design history file is to provide the documentation in parallel with the requirements of 820.30:

a) *design and development plan* (including revisions) -- documented, reviewed, and approved by team;

b) *design input* (also called the requirements document) -- information on intended use, performance, labeling, environment;

c) *design output* -- specifications, top-level drawings, major subassemblies, development of the device master record;

d) *design review* -- minutes, assignments, tracking of issues;

e) *design verification and validation* -- protocols, results of all tests;

f) *design transfer* -- plan for moving into production.

A DHF may be maintained for each design and development activity, by device family or type, or by individual catalog number. A manufacturer may or may not choose to correlate the DHF directly with a 510(k) submission or PMAA.

To assure completion of the record demonstrating that the development plan was followed, an internal audit of the DHF is commonly conducted before the device is released to production.

ACCEPTANCE ACTIVITIES

CHAPTER 9. PURCHASING CONTROLS (SUBPART E)

820.50 PURCHASING CONTROLS

The Requirement

820.50 Purchasing controls. *Each manufacturer shall establish and maintain procedures to ensure that all purchased or otherwise received product and services conform to specified requirements.*

Discussion of the Requirement

The requirements of this section are intended to ensure that purchased, subcontracted, or otherwise received product and services conform to specified requirements and any applicable regulatory requirements. Section 820.3(r) of the regulation defines "product" as "components, manufacturing materials, in-process devices, finished devices, and returned devices." The requirements for purchasing controls apply to all product received from outside by the finished-device manufacturer, including product or services that a manufacturer receives from a "sister facility" or other corporate or financial affiliates.

The manufacturer is expected to establish and maintain documented controls for planning and performing purchasing activities. Controls appropriate to the product or service, and to the effect of the product or service on the quality, safety, and effectiveness of the finished device, are required.

Industry Practice

Manufacturers use various types of procurement quality programs to help ensure that product and contract services, such as testing, calibration, validation, processing, pest control, sterilization, and consulting, will conform to their specified requirements. The most effective purchasing programs promote good working relationships and feedback systems between the supplier and the device manufacturer. An effective purchasing program addresses purchasing requirements/specifications, selection of acceptable suppliers, verification and inspection activities, and required quality records.

820.50(a) EVALUATION OF SUPPLIERS, CONTRACTORS, AND CONSULTANTS

The Requirement

820.50(a) Evaluation of suppliers, contractors, and consultants. *Each manufacturer shall establish and maintain the requirements, including quality requirements, that must be met by suppliers, contractors, and consultants. Each manufacturer shall:*
(1) Evaluate and select potential suppliers, contractors, and consultants on the basis of their ability to meet specified requirements, including quality requirements. The evaluation shall be documented.

(2) Define the type and extent of control to be exercised over the product, services, suppliers, contractors, and consultants, based on the evaluation results.

(3) Establish and maintain records of acceptable suppliers, contractors, and consultants.

Discussion of the Requirement

The Quality System regulation requires manufacturers to ensure the acceptability of purchased, contracted, or otherwise received products and services. This can be accomplished by a combination of documented supplier-implemented quality programs and in-house controls, including the establishment of evaluation criteria, quality requirements, and other requirements, that must be met by the supplier.

Acceptable suppliers, including contractors and consultants, must demonstrate that they are capable of providing products and services that meet these requirements. After suppliers are selected, their performance must be periodically monitored, consistent with the significance of the product or service in question.

While the GMP requirements allow flexibility in determining the degree of assessment and evaluation necessary, manufacturers are required to define the type and extent of control to be exercised over their suppliers. The degree of supplier assurance required will vary with the difficulty of the service, the significance of the product or service, and its potential impact on the performance of the finished device.

Adequate quality system records (QSRs), including records of acceptable suppliers, contractors, and consultants, must be maintained by the manufacturer to demonstrate the capability of suppliers as well as compliance with the requirements of this section. Quality system records such as supplier audit reports and findings will not be reviewed by FDA during routine inspections.

Industry Practice

Manufacturers use various methods to ensure proper evaluation, selection, and control of their suppliers. One of the most common purchasing control systems focuses on the selection, qualification, certification, and approval of suppliers.

General. Evaluating a supplier is an important element of any manufacturer's quality program. Evaluation programs vary depending on the complexity of the product or service supplied, the significance of the product or service, and its possible effect on the effectiveness of the finished device. In general, manufacturers have written procedures in place to describe how product and service specifications will be defined and communicated to suppliers. The procedures typically define items such as

a) methods of supplier evaluation, selection, and control;

b) responsibilities and authority of the manufacturer and supplier;

c) required documentation and data;

d) control and maintenance of documentation and data;

e) communication methods; and

f) the mechanism for control of changes to materials, processes, or specifications.

Procedures for developing purchasing documents usually provide a list of characteristics and requirements that may be relevant when describing products and services.

Specifications. In most instances, manufacturers develop documented specifications for components, packaging, labeling, and the finished product. These documents usually take the form of material specification sheets, drawings, or both. Often, the requirements are initially created during the design control stage. For well-established items, the trade name of the product is often sufficient to describe the material needed. For other items or services, specific written specifications usually are necessary to ensure that the item or service desired is received.

Supplier Evaluation Criteria. Approaches to evaluating potential suppliers vary. One approach is to develop a checklist or matrix that covers quality requirements, design information, documentation system procedures, delivery history, manufacturing process details, part functionality, service availability, reliability, and cost considerations for a given product or service. An interdisciplinary team is identified to establish the qualifying criteria, to review the available data, and to agree on the supplier. The selection team may include representatives from various departments, such as manufacturing, quality assurance, purchasing, and development.

Evaluation criteria for quality requirements may be based on applicable sections of the Quality System regulation, such as design and development, facilities and equipment, materials and components, operations (process capability), finished product, policies and procedures, record-keeping, personnel (education, training, experience), and auditing, depending on the product or service to be supplied. Other minimum requirements that all suppliers are required to meet, such as financial stability and delivery arrangements, also may be determined by the selection team.

The next step is to establish how potential suppliers and contractors will be evaluated. When possible, an evaluation of the supplier's past history in supplying a similar product or service may be performed. Tools such as on-site audits or mail surveys are often used to assess the supplier's quality plan, test and inspection results, validation data, first-article or pilot-run data, history and references, and the results of third-party audits or inspections.

While manufacturers may utilize an existing quality system registration to an ISO 9000 standard as supplier evaluation and selection criteria, they may not necessarily rely on certification as evidence that a supplier has the capability to provide acceptable product or services. Depending on the product or service, an initial assessment or evaluation is typically performed to verify that an adequate quality assurance program is indeed in place.

Where applicable, component samples or first articles are also commonly provided to the manufacturer so that conformance to specifications can be physically verified. Depending on the significance of the purchased item, the evaluation of samples may or may not be coupled with a supplier validation program. The inspection results from the samples or first articles need to be acceptable if the supplier is to be considered further.

When suppliers that meet the evaluation criteria are approved, products or services may be purchased and received. Most manufacturers maintain a list of approved suppliers or equivalent documentation. In addition, documented systems are implemented to ensure that supplier status is verified upon order, including confirmation of the curricula vitae of consultants.

Supplier Relations. After a supplier is chosen and approved, the supplier may be invited to tour the device manufacturer's facility to better understand the end use of the medical device and to review the specification requirements. The manufacturer's ultimate goal is to treat the supplier as an extension of the manufacturer.

Even with a supplier approval program and adequate acceptance activities, manufacturers commonly rely on additional methods for assurance of a supplier's ability to continue to provide an acceptable product or service. The objective is to find the appropriate mixture of assessment tools and incoming inspections and tests necessary for proper control.

For suppliers of major or significant components, initial approval may be followed by an on-site audit of the supplier's facilities. The purpose of the audit is to establish the supplier's ability to conform to the established criteria. Follow-up audits are scheduled on an as-needed basis, dependent on the product or service supplied. Manufacturers often review key component and service suppliers annually and nonsignificant suppliers every 2 to 3 years. When an audit is not feasible or appropriate, the manufacturer may rely on other effective means of ensuring product or service acceptability. Mail surveys in conjunction with the monitoring of receiving quality are often sufficient. All supplier re-audit, survey, and monitoring results are documented and reviewed by the supplier selection team.

Periodic monitoring of ISO certified suppliers may not include on-site assessments or audits, provided that the product or service received continues to meet specified requirements.

Very few manufacturers extend their supplier evaluation and selection programs to include certification, although this process is ultimately the final goal in establishing good working relations with a supplier.

820.50(b) PURCHASING DATA

The Requirement

820.50(b) Purchasing data. Each manufacturer shall establish and maintain data that clearly describe or reference the specified requirements, including quality requirements, for purchased or otherwise received product and services. Purchasing documents shall include, where possible, an agreement that the suppliers, contractors, and consultants agree to notify the manufacturer of changes in the product or service so that manufacturers may determine whether the changes may affect the quality of a finished device. Purchasing data shall be approved in accordance with [section] 820.40.

Discussion of the Requirement

Under the requirements of this section, manufacturers are expected to develop purchasing documents that define specific requirements, including quality requirements, for purchased components, finished devices, packaging materials, labeling materials, manufacturing materials, and contract services. Purchasing specifications for components and product-specific materials are part of the DMR. "Quality requirements" refer to those requirements necessary to ensure that the product or service is adequate for its intended use. The amount of detail required in the purchasing documents relates to the nature of the product or service purchased, taking into account the effect the product or service will have on the safety, effectiveness, and performance of the finished device.

Purchasing data must be provided to the supplier in documents such as, but not limited to, specification sheets, drawings, contracts, or orders. Although documentation may be in a written or electronic media form, in order to ensure that specified requirements are clearly described, manufacturers are required to establish a system for the review and approval of data used to purchase a product or service. The manufacturer is also expected to develop procedures to ensure that requirements are clearly communicated to and understood by the supplier.

It is expected that a manufacturer's purchasing documents will include a statement addressing notification of changes in the supplier's product, process, or service that may affect the performance of the finished device. If the supplier refuses to provide notification, the manufacturer must implement a system of control to ensure that any such changes are identified upon receipt of the material.

Industry Practice

Manufacturers use various methods to describe or reference specifications and quality requirements for their suppliers. Purchasing data can take such forms as standard identification, process instructions, test instructions, and technical information. The information is often communicated to suppliers by means of purchase specifications and/or purchase orders.

Purchasing Specifications. For many items, specifications include a description of the product (e.g., type, grade, class), requirements for material composition and configuration, process instructions (when applicable), performance characteristics and requirements (including references to standards), inspection and test plans, part numbers, requirements for packaging and marking by the supplier, storage and shipping conditions (when required), certifications (e.g., certificates of analysis), requirements for compliance with quality standards (e.g., GMP requirements, ISO standards), and acceptance criteria.

Specifications for services often include reference to regulations and standards. Commonly referenced regulations include the Quality System regulation, the regulation for Good Laboratory Practice for Nonclinical Laboratory Studies (the GLP), and the regulations of the Environmental Protection Agency (EPA) and Occupational Safety and Health Administration (OSHA). Commonly referenced standards include those of AAMI, ISO, ASTM, the Institute of Electrical and Electronics Engineers (IEEE), the U.S. Pharmacopeia (USP), the National Institute for Standards and Technology (NIST), and the Technical Association of the Paper and Pulp Industry (TAPPI). Alternatively, the manufacturer may provide a test method or other internally developed requirement.

If specific process parameters, equipment, tools, and/or supplies are used in the supplier's product or service (e.g., contract sterilization, contract calibration), then these parameters and items are typically documented in a detailed process specification that becomes part of, or is referenced by number in, the manufacturer's contract and/or purchase order.

Purchasing documents are usually established and maintained under a documentation control system to ensure that requirements have been approved and that subsequent changes are evaluated and approved. The document control system typically identifies the individuals who are required to approve documents, describes the records required to demonstrate approval, and defines the distribution, retrieval, and change control system.

Supplier Agreements. Manufacturers typically review the specification requirements with the supplier to ensure that the supplier can provide the product and understands its use in the manufacturer's operation. For standard stock items and minor components, specification review and acceptance by the supplier may not be extensive.

For custom or significant components, finished devices, and services, a formal, written, supplier agreement is more common. Such agreements reference the pertinent specifications, the conditions related to the quality system, environmental requirements (if applicable), financial terms, confidentiality terms, warranties, length of term, and contract responsibilities.

In the case of purchased services, it is common practice for a manufacturer, after discussions with the supplier, to initiate a Request for Service or Proposal, which defines the service requirements and to which the service organization will respond with a contract or letter of understanding. After agreement, the contract is signed by both parties.

Supplier agreements and contracts are typically controlled by the manufacturer's representative responsible for assuring that contract activities are clearly defined and documented. Such contracts are often annually reviewed with the component or service provider to assure that the requirements are still appropriate. Contracts are also reviewed when changes occur to product, processes, services, or other terms.

After the device manufacturer's specifications are generated, the manufacturer's documentation control system is employed to document generation, changes, approval, distribution, and retrieval of obsolete documents.

Purchase Orders. A manufacturer's purchase order typically contains a description of the product or service, the quantity being ordered, the delivery dates, and costs. When placing orders with suppliers of products or services, manufacturers typically refer to specifications, reports, data requirements, and/or contracts on purchase order documents. Some manufacturers include a copy of the related specification(s) with each purchase order.

Purchasing representatives verify that the information presented on purchase orders conforms to approved purchasing documents (e.g., specifications, drawings, contracts) and that the product or service orders are placed only with approved suppliers. These practices are usually documented by standard operating procedures.

Notification of Changes. In many cases, purchase orders contain "boiler-plate" statements requiring suppliers to notify the purchaser when changes are made to the product or service being provided. Because some changes can have a major impact on the performance of the finished device, it is desirable to emphasize this requirement by making it explicit and incorporating a "no change without prior written approval of the purchaser" requirement into the supplier agreement document.

If a supplier does not agree to these terms, and the manufacturer is unable to replace the supplier, increased inspection and testing of incoming materials, on-site supervision when product is being produced, processed, or tested (source inspection), and frequent audits of the supplier are typically performed.

CHAPTER 10. IDENTIFICATION AND TRACEABILITY (SUBPART F)

820.60 IDENTIFICATION

The Requirement

820.60 Identification. *Each manufacturer shall establish and maintain procedures for identifying product during all stages of receipt, production, distribution, and installation to prevent mixups.*

Discussion of the Requirement

Manufacturers are required to establish systems for identification and control of all materials, including components, manufacturing materials, subassemblies, finished devices, packaging, and labeling. These systems must encompass all phases of production, from receipt through distribution and, where applicable, installation.

The purpose of the required controls is to prevent mixups by providing

a) written procedures describing the system(s) used for identification of materials;

b) physical, spatial, or other means of separating incoming, quarantined, accepted, and rejected parts; and,

c) methods of, and controls for, identification of material status.

Industry Practice

Manufacturers use various physical and electronic methods for the identification and control of materials, including tagging, placards, and/or separation.

It is typical for a manufacturer to have a separate physical location (quarantine area) for the holding of uninspected incoming materials. Upon inspection, most manufacturers physically identify materials by status. The most common identification system is color-coded tagging. Segregation may be further enhanced by secure physical separation of parts by their status. Nonconforming materials are typically assigned a final disposition by the material review board (MRB) or similar function.

Identification of parts by status throughout the production process is an important method of ensuring the quality of finished devices. Methods may involve the tagging of parts with a status label, the use of identifying containers, segregation of activities by location, or other means of assuring that only approved parts are used in production.

When tagging methods are utilized, the information identified on the tag varies greatly. Some manufacturers identify only a part number and status. Others include such additional information as lot, batch, or work order identification; quantity; supplier; and (if applicable) waiver number.

Regardless of the methods chosen, written procedures are commonly employed to characterize the methods used and to designate the responsible individuals. These procedures typically define the following elements:

a) assignment of a disposition for all in-coming and in-process materials;

b) identification of the assigned status of all products, including manufacturing materials;

c) method(s) of identification to be used;

d) assignment of designated responsibility for identification activities; and,

e) segregation of unapproved and approved materials.

820.65 TRACEABILITY

The Requirement

820.65 Traceability. Each manufacturer of a device that is intended for surgical implant into the body or to support or sustain life and whose failure to perform when properly used in accordance with instructions for use provided in the labeling can be reasonably expected to result in a significant injury to the user shall establish and maintain procedures for identifying with a control number each unit, lot, or batch of finished devices and where appropriate components. The procedures shall facilitate corrective action. Such identification shall be recorded in the DHR.

Discussion of the Requirement

Manufacturers of products whose failure could result in serious injury or harm to the user are required to establish a documented traceability system. This system must allow for traceability, by control number, of each unit, batch, or lot of finished devices. This requirement also applies to appropriate components of the finished device.

While it is the responsibility of manufacturers to determine if this GMP requirement is applicable to their devices, FDA has indicated that critical devices, as listed in the *Federal Register* notice of March 17, 1988, and *in vitro* diagnostic products are subject to the traceability requirement. In addition, FDA has made it clear that traceability for implantable devices should encompass components and materials used.

Industry Practice

When determining which components and raw materials may be required to be traceable, many manufacturers use the definition of critical components given in the July 21, 1978, version of 21 CFR 820 as guidance. Others perform FMEA or other methods of risk analysis for their products.

Manufacturers use various methods for and levels of traceability, ranging from no traceability to complete traceability of each component to its supplier or raw material lot number. Regardless of the method of traceability utilized for a given device, the extent of traceability, or whether traceability is established for regulatory, liability, or economic reasons, many manufacturers' traceability systems include the following elements:

a) Written procedures describe the control numbering system used, the assignment of control numbers, and how and where control numbers are to be recorded (e.g., in the DHR).

b) Lot numbers, control numbers, or other suitable numbers (e.g., serial numbers for finished devices) are assigned to each lot of components, manufacturing materials, subassemblies, finished devices, packaging, and labeling in order to aid in their identification from the time of receipt forward in the manufacturing process.

c) In-process parts or their containers are physically identified with the assigned lot or control number throughout production.

d) Finished devices are physically identified with the assigned lot, control, or serial number.

e) The assigned lot, control, or serial number is recorded in device distribution records.

When traceability is performed to the component level, it is common practice to assign a control number to each lot of incoming materials. Control numbers, in the form of lot or work order numbers, are also assigned for lower-level operations performed by the manufacturer (e.g., molding or subassembly work). A final control number is assigned to the finished device and is commonly recorded in the distribution record for the device.

CHAPTER 11. RECEIVING, IN-PROCESS, AND FINISHED DEVICE ACCEPTANCE (SUBPART H)

820.80 RECEIVING, IN-PROCESS, AND FINISHED DEVICE ACCEPTANCE

820.80(a) GENERAL

The Requirement

820.80(a) General. Each manufacturer shall establish and maintain procedures for acceptance activities. Acceptance activities include inspections, tests, or other verification activities.

Discussion of the Requirement

This section of the Quality System regulation requires manufacturers to establish and maintain systems and procedures for acceptance activities to verify that all products, including finished devices, work-in-process, components, packaging, labeling, and manufacturing materials, conform to specified requirements. In other words, manufacturers are expected to define the nature and type of acceptance activities required throughout the entire production process to ensure that a given product meets its predetermined quality requirements.

Recognized acceptance activities include, but are not limited to, inspection, test, certificates of analysis, and verification, including supplier audits. While the acceptance activities actually used at different points in the production process may vary, it is expected that manufacturers will determine what activities are necessary and appropriate to assure that specified quality requirements are met.

Industry Practice

Manufacturers recognize that acceptance activities are an integral part of a good quality system but that proper performance of these activities does not, by itself, satisfy the GMP requirements for producing a safe and effective device. Acceptance activities are control methods designed to accept product made according to the manufacturer's specifications. They are intended to prevent further processing or release of a product that does not conform to those specifications. The output of acceptance activities is often used to generate information that may be used in a quality improvement program or to prevent deficiencies or defects in subsequent production of the product.

Historically, most manufacturers implemented "tollgate" systems to test and inspect products at receiving, work-in-process, and finished-device stages to determine their suitability for use. The responsibility for these determinations was typically assigned to the quality control operation. These activities rely on sampling, inspection, and/or testing plans to verify that materials meet established criteria for physical characteristics and performance after processing operations are concluded.

It is recognized that there are serious shortcomings to "tollgate" inspection operations. The most significant shortcoming of this traditional method of product acceptance is that it is performed too late to prevent costly and time-consuming material or product quality problems. With the increasing use of "just-in-time" and similar manufacturing systems and with continually evolving product quality, price, and delivery competition in the global marketplace, larger demands have been placed on traditional quality-control materials inspection, test, and acceptance activities.

In this changing environment, manufacturers recognize that traditional methods of manufacturing, inspection, and test may not meet the increasing need to be more time- and cost-effective. Many progressive manufacturers have developed their inspection, test, and verification activities with the intention of preventing material or product quality problems. In addition, newly developed acceptance techniques provide improved methods of demonstrating that processes and products meet specifications. The advantage of such systems is that manufacturers are able to act on quality issues early in the manufacturing process, before operations are completed and severe difficulties are encountered. Many of these tools continuously monitor identified programs for compliance, so that noncompliances and other concerns are identified, addressed, and corrected before manufacturing activities begin.

These progressive techniques not only meet the requirements set forth in the regulation, but accomplish this goal effectively and with efficiency and cost containment. Manufacturers who rely on prevention techniques are able to recognize and solve product quality problems much earlier in the product design or manufacturing cycle, thus lowering the quality costs related to product complaints, rework, scrap, and downtime.

Effective acceptance procedures and systems directly affect the ability of a manufacturer to demonstrate that processes and product meet specifications. These procedures and systems are developed during the design stage and undergo the same design reviews as do product and process designs.

820.80(b) RECEIVING ACCEPTANCE ACTIVITIES

The Requirement

820.80(b) Receiving acceptance activities. Each manufacturer shall establish and maintain procedures for acceptance of incoming product. Incoming product shall be inspected, tested, or otherwise verified as conforming to specified requirements. Acceptance or rejection shall be documented.

Discussion of the Requirement

Each manufacturer is expected to establish an effective receiving acceptance program for all product coming into the facility. The program must ensure that product arriving at the receiving dock is or has been properly inspected, tested, evaluated, or verified to determine whether it meets defined specifications. This evaluation results in a documented decision to accept or reject the product. The program also must describe, and require documentation of, the methods used to release product for further processing. All parts, components, and materials that will become part of the finished device or part of the manufacturing materials used in the processing of the device must go through a receiving acceptance process. This does not necessarily mean that each lot, batch, or item has to be inspected and tested by the device manufacturer, but there must be a defined method of evaluating whether that lot, batch, or item meets its predetermined quality requirements.

The FDA has noted that manufacturers are permitted to release for "urgent use" incoming items that have not yet been proven to be acceptable for use, provided that control of the unapproved item is maintained and that the manufacturer can retrieve product containing the item *before* distribution. The FDA does not permit the distribution of unapproved finished devices based on the "urgent use" provision.

Industry Practice

Most manufacturers have established receiving inspection or incoming inspection organizations that are responsible for receiving acceptance activities. Typically, an SOP is created to describe the overall process, which may involve source inspection programs, supplier audit and/or certification programs, test and inspection programs, or a combination of these and other methods.

Additional SOPs are sometimes created to describe the process in greater detail (e.g., dock-to-stock programs). Supplemental documents are usually generated to describe the inspection and test requirements for specific products being processed. These documents may describe measurements to be made or tests to be run, any required instruments or gauges, sampling plans for each characteristic to be evaluated, and the records necessary to document designated activities and results. Additional special requirements, such as outside laboratory tests, certificates of analysis, or certificates of compliance, may be described in these or other documents. Test procedures and test stations/methods are validated, and each test setup is documented. All measuring equipment is under calibration control in accordance with section 820.72.

Inspection/test results are typically recorded in a manner that facilitates review and analysis of the quality performance and quality variances of the supplied product. Many manufacturers recognize that the results of analysis of quantitative test data are more useful than the analysis of "pass/fail" data and therefore require that quantitative measurements be recorded for future review. The data generated are used to monitor product and supplier performance trends. Quality system data review and analysis provide opportunities for improvement and permit timely changes to be made in the acceptance criteria, methods, or procedures for the product. For example, surveillance may be increased if performance is slipping below norm or reduced if performance is exceeding expectation. Quality system data review and analysis also provide feedback to suppliers so that supplier-related deficiencies can be detected and corrected before the next shipment. Conversely, good performance may result in a certification process or the implementation of some form of "skip-lot" or dock-to-stock program for particular suppliers.

The documented receiving data generally include

a) the date of the inspection;

b) the part number or other unique product configuration identifier;

c) the lot, batch, or serial number identification provided by the supplier;

d) a supplemental control number if the supplier identification is insufficient or incompatible with the manufacturer's method of recording this information (or if, as per section 820.65, a control number is required for the protection of the public health);

e) the quantity received;

f) the quantity inspected/tested;

g) numerical test results;

h) the quantity of pass/fail items in the sample;

i) the quantity of lot/batch rejected; and,

j) other pertinent information concerning disposition or special events surrounding the acceptance process.

Controls are usually implemented to ensure that product that has not yet been inspected/tested is quarantined and that rejected product is quarantined and properly dispositioned. Not all manufacturers allow release of incoming items for "urgent use," although this practice is becoming more common. Where this practice is permitted, documented systems are developed to ensure that proper controls are in place. In addition to material identification, these systems include mechanisms to prevent product from being released for distribution before successful completion of the receiving acceptance activity, which is often tied into the finished-device record review process.

820.80(c) IN-PROCESS ACCEPTANCE ACTIVITIES

The Requirement

820.80(c) In-process acceptance activities. Each manufacturer shall establish and maintain acceptance procedures, where appropriate, to ensure that specified requirements for in-process product are met. Such procedures shall ensure that in-process product is controlled until the required inspection and tests or other verification activities have been completed, or necessary approvals are received, and are documented.

Discussion of the Requirement

When appropriate and feasible, in-process acceptance activities are performed at appropriate points in the process to ensure that any in-process quality requirements have been met. These acceptance activities must be performed according to written procedures that include, but are not limited to, descriptions of the necessary equipment, required methods, and acceptance criteria. Similar to the requirements for incoming items, manufacturers can use product, under defined, documented conditions, before all in-process acceptance activities have been completed. However, these activities must be completed *before* the product is released for distribution. When in-process acceptance activities are performed, they must be documented.

Industry Practice

In general, the purpose of in-process acceptance activities is to verify that defined quality requirements for in-process products are met. In-process acceptance activities typically also allow early detection of nonconformances, preventing further processing of nonconforming items, increasing the probability of producing a finished device that meets specifications, and improving the efficiency of the entire operation.

In-process acceptance activities usually include quality control tests that yield quantitative measurements (e.g., weights, flows, pressures, pH, viscosity, porosity, voltage, resistance). Visual inspections and tests that supply only "go/no-go" results are also performed. For example, visual inspection of circuit boards for solder integrity is an in-process visual inspection. Automated circuit board testing is also performed, and "passed" or "failed" results are documented.

The "appropriateness" of the points at which in-process acceptance activities are performed depends on a number of factors, including the extent of process validation, the complexity of the manufacturing process, and the in-process material characteristics that can change with time or be affected by previous and subsequent processes. Similarly, the extent to which in-process acceptance activities must be performed depends on the type, complexity, and number of processes involved in the manufacturing of the device. In-process acceptance activities may involve sampling according to a statistically valid plan; testing the beginning, middle, and end of a batch; or performing a setup inspection of an automated system.

Manufacturers typically document the results of in-process acceptance activities on prepared forms or test records that are included in the product's DHR. Results also may be recorded in engineering notebooks or production forms that are more universal in their application. The DHR package either contains copies of these records or references the location of the documents. The documentation includes the date and the results; and the person who performed the activity typically stamps, signs, or initials the record to document that the activity was performed.

In-process data also may be recorded on some type of statistical process quality control chart (e.g., a precontrol or "rainbow" chart, an "X Bar" chart, an "R" chart). These charts are used to monitor the variability of the process. If trends are seen, appropriate investigations are generally performed and corrective action is taken.

Most manufacturers assign in-process acceptance activities either to the production department or the quality department. An independent review of documented results is commonly performed to ensure that the acceptance activity was performed correctly and that the in-process product meets the specified criteria. For this purpose, the quality function may review or audit the results recorded by production, or a routine audit of acceptance activities may be performed and documented by the quality function.

Many manufacturers place in-process materials in an area designated as "quarantined" until the results of in-process acceptance activities are obtained and reviewed. Other common methods include the use of tags, colored stickers, computer labels, or other systems, as per section 820.86.

Because any in-process failures must be documented and the in-process material dispositioned accordingly (e.g., reworked, scrapped, or "used as is"), many firms use a type of nonconformance system when in-process failures occur. The results are reviewed by a designated person or group, such as an MRB, to determine the final disposition of the material, which is generally documented by means of a nonconformance report or similar mechanism. This report is then filed or referenced in the DHR. This mechanism is particularly significant in those cases where the disposition is "use as is," as it is a means of documenting a valid reason for such a disposition. When a rework is possible (i.e., when reworking will not adversely affect the material in any way), this mechanism ensures that reworked material is reevaluated to determine whether it meets specifications.

The number and types of in-process test failures are typically included in the evaluation of the adequacy of the firm's QA program. Documenting actual quantitative test results, when possible, will provide more information for quality review and corrective action.

820.80(d) FINAL ACCEPTANCE ACTIVITIES

The Requirement

820.80 (d) Final acceptance activities. Each manufacturer shall establish and maintain procedures for finished device acceptance to ensure that each production run, lot, or batch of finished devices meets acceptance criteria. Finished devices shall be held in quarantine or otherwise adequately controlled until released. Finished devices shall not be released for distribution until: (1) The activities required in the DMR are completed; (2) the associated data and documentation is reviewed; (3) the release is authorized by the signature of a designated individual(s); and (4) the authorization is dated.

Discussion of the Requirement

Manufacturers are expected to establish procedures that define the acceptance activities required for each production run, lot, or batch of finished devices. These procedures should include, but are not limited to, descriptions of any equipment required, the methods used to perform the activity, and the acceptance criteria. Some information, such as the acceptance criteria, may be in other DMR documents. All finished devices awaiting review or undergoing review must be prevented from being distributed until released.

Finished-device acceptance activities also must include a review of the DHR to ensure that all processing steps were performed and completed in accordance with the DMR. This review must be performed by a designated individual, and the results of the review must be documented, including the authorizing individual's signature and the date.

Industry Practice

Finished-device-acceptance activities augment the acceptance activities performed during processing and ensure that all manufacturing and packaging processes have been performed correctly. Finished-device acceptance activities may include the use of a statistically valid sampling plan to test and inspect units from each lot or batch. In accordance with section 820.170, finished devices that are installed or assembled on-site are required to be verified after installation. Finished-device acceptance activities increase the probability of producing a finished product that meets specifications.

The extent and type of finished-device acceptance activities performed generally depends on the complexity of the device and on the type, complexity, and number of processes involved in the manufacturing of the device. Other factors may include the type of in-process acceptance activities performed and the extent and adequacy of any process validations. In other words, how much "up-front" control has been implemented? Where possible, finished-device acceptance activities commonly simulate actual conditions of use. Most manufacturers require some type of quantitative test results as part of the finished-device performance testing program (e.g., weights, flows, pressures, pH, viscosity, porosity, voltage, resistance).

Most quality testing and inspection responsibilities, including finished-device testing, are assigned to QA personnel. Production personnel are sometimes responsible for performing finished-device testing and/or inspection, and the results are reviewed by QA personnel to ensure that the testing was performed correctly and that finished products met the specified criteria. In addition, QA personnel may retest a few finished units as an audit of the product and the final-test process.

Manufacturers commonly document the results of finished-device acceptance activities in the DHR. Results also may be recorded on other forms or in engineering notebooks. The DHR package either contains copies of these records or references the location of the documents. The documentation includes the test results and the date; and the person who performed the acceptance activity stamps, signs, or initials the record to document that the activity was performed.

Because finished devices need to be appropriately identified and quarantined to prevent their use until they have been accepted, many manufacturers place finished devices in an area designated as "quarantined" until the results of final acceptance activities are obtained and the DHR record has been reviewed. Other common methods include the use of tags, colored stickers, computer labels, or identification systems, as per sections 820.60 and 820.86.

Because any finished-device failures should be documented and the finished device dispositioned accordingly (e.g., reworked, scrapped, or "used as is"), many manufacturers use a type of nonconformance system when in-process failures occur. As part of the overall quality system, such a system allows prompt investigations of finished products, packaging, and labeling that do not meet finished-device acceptance criteria. The results are reviewed by a designated person or group of personnel, such as an MRB, to determine the final disposition of the material, which is documented by means of a nonconformance report or similar mechanism and then filed with the DHR. This mechanism is particularly significant in those cases where the disposition is "use as is," because it is a means of documenting a valid reason for such a disposition. When a rework decision is possible (i.e., when reworking does not adversely affect the finished product), this mechanism ensures that the reworked device is reevaluated to confirm that it meets specifications. When a "scrap" disposition is made, this mechanism provides a convenient means of documenting the decision.

The number and types of finished-device failures are typically reviewed during the evaluation of the adequacy of the manufacturer's QA program, an activity made even more important by the new GMP requirements. Documenting actual quantitative test results, when possible, will provide more information for quality review.

820.80(e) ACCEPTANCE RECORDS

The Requirement

820.80 (e) Acceptance records. Each manufacturer shall document acceptance activities required by this part. These records shall include: (1) The acceptance activities performed; (2) the dates acceptance activities are performed; (3) the results; (4) the signature of the individual(s) conducting the acceptance activities; and (5) where appropriate the equipment used. These records shall be part of the DHR.

Discussion of the Requirement

All receiving, in-process, and final acceptance activities must be recorded. Requirements for the associated records are spelled out in the regulation. Manufacturers are expected to have records that show that a stated acceptance activity was performed and whether the product passed or failed that activity. Each manufacturer also must determine when to identify the equipment used for the acceptance activity. It is strongly recommended that manufacturers record quantitative data if it is generated. Equipment identification should be recorded when deemed necessary for proper investigations into nonconforming product.

Industry Practice

Common record-keeping practices used by manufacturers are detailed in the "Industry Practice" portions of sections 820.80(b), 820.80(c), and 820.80(d).

CHAPTER 12. ACCEPTANCE STATUS (SUBPART H)

820.86 ACCEPTANCE STATUS

The Requirement

820.86 Acceptance status. Each manufacturer shall identify by suitable means the acceptance status of product, to indicate the conformance or nonconformance of product with acceptance criteria. The identification of acceptance status shall be maintained throughout manufacturing, packaging, labeling, installation, and servicing of the product to ensure that only product which has passed the required acceptance activities is distributed, used, or installed.

Discussion of the Requirement

The intent of this requirement is to minimize opportunities for mixups of acceptable and unacceptable product by requiring that the acceptance status be clearly identified. Systems developed to meet the requirements of section 820.60, "Identification," also may be used to help show the acceptance status required by section 820.86.

It must be possible to quickly and clearly establish the inspection status of product at any phase of the activities carried out during receiving, production, storage, holding, installation, and servicing. This is especially important for those items that have been determined not to conform to acceptance requirements. The requirement is also applicable to servicing; therefore, devices awaiting service and those that have been serviced already must be identified as to their acceptance status.

Industry Practice

Industry currently utilizes both physical and electronic methods for identifying the acceptance status of product. Acceptance status may be indicated physically or electronically by labels, tags, stickers, signatures, bar codes, or other means. For example, the acceptance status of product is commonly identified with "accept" or "reject" labels, stamps, or stickers. "Accept" labels may be green; "reject" labels are typically red to provide a clear indication of the product status. Some manufacturers indicate the acceptance status of incoming, in-process, and finished product by means of a traveler or history card that accompanies the product as it is moved from station to station. When these identifiers are used, they are displayed so that the status is readily visible to prevent inadvertent moving or use of product that is in quarantine.

A number of device manufacturers use computer systems to control released product in warehouses and product awaiting incoming acceptance. Product status is identified in a computer, and product is picked automatically for release or other disposition. In accordance with the GMP requirement, many manufacturers already have validated these systems.

Basically, any means may be used to indicate the acceptance status, provided that it is proven to be effective. However, if the method used results in mixups of acceptable and unacceptable product, then in all likelihood the method will be challenged by FDA. The identification method chosen indicates the status of the product with respect to whether it has been inspected/tested and accepted, rejected, or placed on hold awaiting disposition.

CHAPTER 13. STATISTICAL TECHNIQUES (SUBPART O)

820.250 STATISTICAL TECHNIQUES

The Requirement

820.250 Statistical techniques.

(a) Where appropriate, each manufacturer shall establish and maintain procedures for identifying valid statistical techniques required for establishing, controlling, and verifying the acceptability of process capability and product characteristics.

(b) Sampling plans, when used, shall be written and based on a valid statistical rationale. Each manufacturer shall establish and maintain procedures to ensure that sampling methods are adequate for their intended use and to ensure that when changes occur the sampling plans are reviewed. These activities shall be documented.

Discussion of the Requirement

The requirements of this section apply throughout the design process, production, and the evaluation of post-distribution data. Elsewhere in the Quality System regulation, only three references are made to statistical techniques (sampling plans, service reports, and quality problems). However, manufacturers are expected to use valid statistical methodologies whenever appropriate.

The actual techniques and methods used are left to the discretion of the manufacturer; however, the methodology must be capable of withstanding statistical scrutiny. It is implied that when statistical tools are used to analyze quality data, baseline, alert, and action threshold levels should be established, reviewed, and revised on a regular basis.

In addition, device manufacturers must establish and maintain procedures to ensure that any sampling methods used are appropriate for their intended use and are regularly reviewed. The sampling plans selected must be adequate to ensure that unacceptable product quality is detected. If the quality goals of the manufacturer, suppliers, or users change, it will be necessary to select a different sampling plan. When more units of product of unacceptable quality are detected than are allowed by the selected sampling plan, the associated manufacturing processes must be adjusted.

Industry Practice

It is common for manufacturers to utilize statistical methods throughout the life cycle of a device. These techniques are incorporated into the design phase, carried though production, and used in the analysis of post-distribution quality data. They are beneficial in a wide variety of circumstances, including data collection, analysis, and application. Appropriate statistical techniques can assist the manufacturer not only in deciding what data to obtain, but also in making the best use of the data.

Manufacturers use statistical techniques during design to conduct market analysis and estimate reliability, maintainability, shelf life, and risk level. In production, these techniques are usually applied to demonstrate process capability and product conformance to specified requirements.

Statistical methods are also commonly used for

a) product and process limit determination;
b) defect rate estimation;
c) process control;
d) sampling plan and quality level determination;
e) sampling;
f) nonconformity analysis;
g) risk determination;
h) root causes determination;
i) data assessment; and
j) verification and measurement.

Commonly used statistical methods include pareto charts, histograms, control charts, design of experiment, regression analysis, and analysis of variance. For purposes of sampling, inspection, and test, many manufacturers rely on published sampling plans recognized by FDA (e.g., ANSI/ASQC Z1.4). However, an increasing number of companies are developing their own sampling plans in order to evaluate processes and product efficiently and effectively.

PRODUCTION AND PROCESS CONTROL

CHAPTER 14. PRODUCTION AND PROCESS CONTROLS (SUBPART G)

820.70 PRODUCTION AND PROCESS CONTROLS

820.70(a) GENERAL

The Requirement

820.70 Production and process controls.

(a) *General.* Each manufacturer shall develop, conduct, control, and monitor production processes to ensure that a device conforms to its specifications. Where deviations from device specifications could occur as a result of the manufacturing process, the manufacturer shall establish and maintain process control procedures that describe any process controls necessary to ensure conformance to specifications. Where process controls are needed, they shall include:

(1) Documented instructions, standard operating procedures (SOP's), and methods that define and control the manner of production;

(2) Monitoring and control of process parameters and component and device characteristics during production;

(3) Compliance with specified reference standards or codes;

(4) The approval of processes and process equipment; and

(5) Criteria for workmanship which shall be expressed in documented standards or by means of identified and approved representative samples.

Discussion of the Requirement

The objective of this GMP requirement is to ensure that each manufacturer produces devices that conform to specification, as defined and approved during the design phase. It is each manufacturer's responsibility to evaluate manufacturing processes to determine if the lack of process controls could affect the reliability and repeatability of the manufacturing process. If it is determined that process controls are required, these controls must be established, implemented, monitored, and verified to the degree necessary to prevent product nonconformance. The generation of procedures is necessary to ensure consistency in manufacture. Process controls include standards, production methods and instructions, procedures, workmanship criteria, drawings, process validation, inspection, testing, and evaluation.

The controlled process must be monitored to ensure that it remains in control. Documented evidence of the monitoring of process parameters and device/component characteristics is expected. The documentation should identify the equipment used, the operating conditions, and the personnel performing activities. When the process is observed to be out of control, appropriate action is expected to be taken to evaluate the product and the continuation of the process.

If it is determined that a process does not have an impact on product quality and thus does not require process controls, there must be a documented rationale with an approval date and the signature of the responsible authority.

Industry Practice

Device manufacturers document procedures and process specifications, describing the manner of production and, when deemed necessary, process controls.

Typically, manufacturers begin in the design phase to develop the manufacturing process based on product design, materials and components, and quality characteristics required. The development of the manufacturing process often involves assessment of the environment, the required utilities, the skill requirements for personnel, and the compatibility of materials with equipment. Device complexity is a determining factor in process controls. Some processes are simple assembly operations, while others may require soldering, grinding, or plating. Still other processes are yet more complex, such as aseptic filling or sterilization. The characteristics of the device define the process and the required process controls.

Processes that often require process controls include, but are not limited to, sterilization, aseptic filling, cleaning, soldering, electroplating, mixing, injection molding, package sealing, water systems, heat treating, and heating, ventilation, and air conditioning (HVAC) systems.

Manufacturers typically conduct process validation, which may include equipment installation qualification, equipment operational qualification, and process performance qualification. Protocols are written, approved, and implemented. Upon completion of each activity, a report is issued regarding the outcome of the qualification. Based upon these activities, documented instructions (e.g., procedures, process specifications, routers, drawings) are developed for routine production. These documents commonly identify

    a) process conditions, including accepted variances;

    b) types of equipment and instruments required;

    c) responsibilities for operating, controlling, monitoring, and approving the process;

    d) frequency of monitoring;

    e) instructions (e.g., steps, sequence, start-up requirements, required checks);

    f) requirements for requalification;

    g) materials required;

    h) criteria for workmanship (e.g., drawings, master samples, test methods, limits);

    i) process control indicators (e.g., dosimeters, biological indicators, metal detector standards, gauges, dials);

    j) environmental conditions, when required; and,

    k) documentation requirements.

To support the operation, programs for preventive maintenance, calibration, and employee training/ certification, as required, are established.

820.70(b) PRODUCTION AND PROCESS CHANGES

The Requirement

820.70(b) **Production and process changes.** *Each manufacturer shall establish and maintain procedures for changes to a specification, method, process, or procedure. Such changes shall be verified or where appropriate validated according to [section] 820.75, before implementation and these activities shall be documented. Changes shall be approved in accordance with [section] 820.40.*

Discussion of the Requirement

Each manufacturer is required to establish and maintain procedures for changes to any requirement with which a product, process, service, or other activity must comply. Changes must be subject to controls as stringent as those applied to the original specification, method, process, or procedure. Prior to approval and implementation, the change must be verified or, if determined necessary, validated in accordance with section 820.75, "Process validation."

Approved changes must be communicated to the appropriate personnel (e.g., line operators, supervisors, suppliers, sterilizer operators, purchasing personnel) in a timely manner to allow for implementation and, if necessary, training.

Industry Practice

It is common for manufacturers to develop one program that is utilized for all documents and changes (see Chapter 23). When a single program is used, changes are typically classified by type (e.g., specification, procedure, process), since production and process changes may require a more detailed evaluation and approval, including verification or validation, than other document changes.

820.70(c) ENVIRONMENTAL CONTROL

The Requirement

820.70(c) **Environmental control.** *Where environmental conditions could reasonably be expected to have an adverse effect on product quality, the manufacturer shall establish and maintain procedures to adequately control these environmental conditions. Environmental control system(s) shall be periodically inspected to verify that the system, including necessary equipment, is adequate and functioning properly. These activities shall be documented and reviewed.*

Discussion of the Requirement

The objective of this GMP requirement is to ensure that environmental conditions that could have an adverse effect on product quality are controlled. Each manufacturer is expected to evaluate the environment in which components, manufacturing materials, packaging, labeling, and in-process, finished, and returned devices are manufactured and held to determine what, if any, environmental controls are necessary. The degree of environmental control must be consistent with the intended use of the device.

Requirements for environmental controls must be defined and documented. In addition, written procedures are required to ensure control of conditions and periodic inspection of the control systems. This inspection must include any applicable equipment (e.g., pumps, filters, measurement equipment).

Industry Practice

Manufacturers maintain environmental controls commensurate with the product being manufactured and the function of a given manufacturing or storage area. Conditions that are routinely considered for control include lighting, ventilation, temperature, humidity, air pressure, air flow, filtration, airborne contamination, microbial contamination, and electrostatic discharge (ESD).

Industry practices related to the control of the environment vary from comprehensive clean-room controls for the production of sterile and aseptic products, to the control of ESD for the manufacture of products that contain microcircuits or that may be damaged by ESD, to general control of particulates, humidity, and temperature.

The degree of control for any given environmental element may also vary within a given facility. For example, ESD controls can range from a combination of protective packaging, grounded wrist straps, and conductive work surfaces to the combined use of protective packaging, conductive holding fixtures, grounded wrist straps, floor mats, antistatic clothing, conductive work surfaces, ionized air blowers, and conductive chairs, floors, shoes, carriers, and storage shelves. The controls necessary and the effectiveness of ESD controls installed are determined as part of the validation of the process or activity. Consideration of ESD controls includes evaluation of manufacturing processes such as packaging, molding, and other activities that may generate damaging electrical charges.

Written procedures are typically developed to define the environmental conditions being controlled. These procedures may encompass

 a) the elements to be controlled;
 b) the areas affected;
 c) environmental specifications and action limits;
 d) the types and locations of controls;
 e) the method(s) of monitoring;

f) the frequency of inspection intervals;

g) the frequency of calibration intervals (if applicable);

h) procedures for corrective action;

i) documentation requirements; and,

j) training requirements (if applicable).

Examples of control-system inspection activities include particle count tests, calibration of control instrumentation, and the review of strip charts for temperature and relative humidity measurements. The inspection and review of environmental control systems are usually part of the production QA program.

820.70(d) PERSONNEL

The Requirement

820.70(d) Personnel. Each manufacturer shall establish and maintain requirements for the health, cleanliness, personal practices, and clothing of personnel if contact between such personnel and product or environment could reasonably be expected to have an adverse effect on product quality. The manufacturer shall ensure that maintenance and other personnel who are required to work temporarily under special environmental conditions are appropriately trained or supervised by a trained individual.

Discussion of the Requirement

Manufacturers must define requirements and establish written procedures when unclean or inappropriately dressed employees, or employees with medical conditions, could adversely affect the quality of the product. Manufacturers must determine and document the requirements for acceptable clothing (e.g., clean dress, smocks, coveralls, masks, gowns, head covering, beard covering, gloves, safety apparel), hygiene (handwashing and toilet facilities), and personnel practices (e.g., eating, drinking, smoking) applicable to the device being manufactured.

Requirements for sterile devices and clean-room or environmentally-controlled-room operations may necessitate a higher level of control in order to minimize the bioburden or particulate contamination of the device and the contamination of the environment. Each manufacturer must evaluate the extent of cleanliness required based upon device cleaning procedures, aseptic operations, and/or terminal sterilization.

It is expected that all personnel working under special environmental conditions will be trained in the requirements for working in those areas, including requirements for hygiene, health, dress, cleanliness, personal practices, and notification of supervisors of activities. Manufacturers are also required to define and document requirements for temporary personnel, such as maintenance, cleaning, and temporary employees. The requirements may include appropriate training of such personnel and/or direct supervision by a trained individual.

Industry Practice

Manufacturers typically establish and document in their quality systems some basic requirements for personnel with regard to dress codes and cleanliness, and they provide designated areas, separate from production and laboratory operations, for eating, drinking, and smoking. Applicable procedures commonly include

    a) required attire;
    b) manufacturing areas affected;
    c) entry and exit gowning practices;
    d) handling of adverse medical conditions; and,
    e) training requirements.

Nonsterile Devices. For the manufacture of nonsterile devices, clean everyday attire is usually adequate. In operations such as machine shops, clean everyday attire also may be adequate if the device will be cleaned and controlled in later stages of manufacture. Many manufacturers provide uniforms and/or labcoats to personnel for use on the premises, if deemed necessary.

Sterile Devices. For sterile devices, aseptic operations, and some electronic devices, the requirements become more specific. The requirements are determined based upon impact on product quality, whether it be bioburden levels, particulate contamination, or sterility assurance. However, the requirements may vary depending on downstream processing.

Dress codes are commonly mandated for clean-room or environmentally-controlled-room operations. Required attire typically includes head coverings, beard and mustache covers, gowns or coveralls, masks, and shoe coverings.

Procedures for the reporting of medical conditions (e.g., coughing, sneezing, lesions or sores, conjunctivitis) are important in these areas and for these products, since there are potential effects on product quality and/or the environment. Personnel report such conditions to their supervisor, who evaluates the impact on activities. Often, personnel are assigned different tasks until they are well.

Manufacturers provide specialized training to all personnel working under special environmental conditions. The level of training may be different for nonproduction/QA personnel than for temporary employees. In the absence of training, direct supervision is provided.

820.70(e) CONTAMINATION CONTROL

The Requirement

820.70(e) Contamination control. Each manufacturer shall establish and maintain procedures to prevent contamination of equipment or product by substances that could reasonably be expected to have an adverse effect on product quality.

Discussion of the Requirement

Each manufacturer must establish and maintain procedures to prevent contamination of equipment, components, manufacturing materials, in-process devices, finished devices, and returned devices by substances that could adversely affect device safety or effectiveness. There must be periodic, documented checks or inspections to verify that the contamination control system is properly functioning.

The system must include adequate cleaning procedures and schedules if such controls are necessary to meet manufacturing specifications. Sewage, trash, byproducts, chemical effluvium, and other refuse that could adversely affect a device's quality also must be adequately controlled.

Industry Practice

Manufacturers typically establish and document basic contamination control requirements within the quality system. The following are common elements of a contamination control program:

a) cleaning and sanitation procedures and schedules necessary to meet manufacturing specifications, such as procedures addressing personnel cleanliness, the adequacy of washing and toilet facilities, personnel dress codes, and designated areas for eating, drinking, and smoking;

b) procedures designed to prevent contamination of equipment, components, or finished devices by rodenticides, insecticides, fungicides, fumigants, other cleaning and sanitation substances, and hazardous substances; and,

c) procedures for handling sewage, byproducts, chemical effluents, and other refuse of the manufacturing process in a timely, safe, and sanitary manner.

Manufacturers typically establish general cleaning and sanitation procedures and schedules for all areas (e.g., manufacturing, personnel support areas) to ensure a clean working environment for all employees. There are usually separate procedures and schedules for areas requiring special environmental conditions. In these areas, dress codes and other special requirements are posted so that all personnel are notified of the restrictions.

Contamination control procedures for rodenticides, insecticides, fungicides, fumigants, hazardous substances, and the like are typically handled by the maintenance department for the entire facility. Outside contractors may be consulted as needed.

Procedures for cleaning, sanitation, and other contamination control measures typically address

a) affected areas and locations;
b) materials and chemicals to be utilized;
c) special instructions or precautions;

d) applicable contracts, when necessary;

e) documentation requirements; and,

f) applicable schedules, when required.

820.70(f) BUILDINGS

The Requirement

820.70(f) Buildings. *Buildings shall be of suitable design and contain sufficient space to perform necessary operations, prevent mixups, and assure orderly handling.*

Discussion of the Requirement

The manufacturer is responsible for evaluating the manufacturing facility to ensure that the building, utilities, and space allow for proper product and area identification and for the performance of necessary manufacturing and associated functions. The manufacturer is responsible for providing adequate space to prevent mixups and assure orderly handling of

a) incoming components;

b) rejected or obsolete products/components;

c) in-process products/components;

d) finished product/components;

e) labeling;

f) product/components that have been reprocessed, repaired, or reworked;

g) equipment, drawings, blueprints, tools, molds, patterns, records;

h) testing and laboratory operations; and,

i) quarantined product/components.

Industry Practice

Manufacturers ordinarily put together a floor plan establishing the flow of product and designating receiving areas, areas for acceptable and rejected product/components, manufacturing areas, storage areas for components/product and finished goods, rework/reprocessing/repair areas, office space, and nonmanufacturing areas (e.g., cafeterias, restrooms). This approach enables management to plan growth, locate personnel support functions close to the areas affected, and eliminate excessive handling of product/components and finished goods during the manufacturing process.

820.70(g) EQUIPMENT

The Requirement

820.70(g) Equipment. Each manufacturer shall ensure that all equipment used in the manufacturing process meets specified requirements and is appropriately designed, constructed, placed, and installed to facilitate maintenance, adjustment, cleaning, and use.

(1) Maintenance schedule. Each manufacturer shall establish and maintain schedules for the adjustment, cleaning, and other maintenance of equipment to ensure that manufacturing specifications are met. Maintenance activities, including the date and individual(s) performing the maintenance activities, shall be documented.

(2) Inspection. Each manufacturer shall conduct periodic inspections in accordance with established procedures to ensure adherence to applicable equipment maintenance schedules. The inspections, including the date and individual(s) conducting the inspections, shall be documented.

(3) Adjustment. Each manufacturer shall ensure that any inherent limitations or allowable tolerances are visibly posted on or near equipment requiring periodic adjustments or are readily available to personnel performing these adjustments.

Discussion of the Requirement

Section 820.70(g) requires manufacturers to ensure that all equipment (e.g., fabrication, molding, extrusion, assembly, packaging, sterilization) is appropriately designed and installed to facilitate maintenance, adjustment, cleaning, and use. Equipment must also meet the requirements that are necessary to ensure its proper functioning in the manufacture of the device.

A maintenance schedule must be developed if a manufacturer determines that maintenance is required on a particular piece of equipment. The schedule must be available to designated individuals who operate and maintain the equipment. Records must be maintained for each piece of equipment, documenting the maintenance activities performed and including the signature of the person who performed the activities. This requirement applies to maintenance performed by both internal and external resources.

When maintenance activity is required, the manufacturer must document and follow procedures for inspection of maintenance activities to ensure that such activity is conducted according to schedule, that all activities have been completed, and that equipment specification requirements continue to be met. Records must be maintained of maintenance activity inspections, including the date of the inspection and the name of the person who conducted the inspection. Inspection findings must be reviewed by management and corrective/preventive action taken as appropriate.

If adjustments are required to maintain equipment operation, the limits and tolerances must be documented and made available to those individuals responsible for making the adjustments (i.e., operators, maintenance personnel). This information can be provided as an approved document posted on the equipment or located nearby in the work area.

Industry Practice

Manufacturers typically prepare equipment specifications based upon needs identified during the design phase. When required, installation and operational qualification protocols are commonly developed and documented for each piece of equipment to ensure that it meets specification and functions in the intended manner. The qualification activities includes verification of all parts, functions, codes, and utilities; the establishment of cleaning, maintenance, and (when required) calibration methods; and, operational performance testing.

Maintenance procedures and schedules are developed by manufacturers to maintain equipment operation and reduce the risk of major repair and service. The initial maintenance activities are often based on information provided in equipment operating or maintenance manuals. Typically, a schedule is developed that identifies each piece of equipment, the maintenance activity required, the maintenance methods to be used, and the frequency of maintenance. This information is often documented in a master schedule and/or card file system with supporting maintenance forms that provide instructions and also serve as records of activities. Many manufacturers use off-the-shelf software programs to document and manage the maintenance program. These software programs often provide formats for master schedules, work orders, records, and reports.

Records of maintenance activities commonly include the date(s) of service, the service performed, and the signature of the individual who performed the activity. In most cases, maintenance records are reviewed for completeness and conformance by the maintenance supervisor/manager/lead and are signed and dated by that designated individual. When maintenance activity is performed by outside contractors, the manufacturer most often maintains the schedule and identifies the activities to be performed. The contractor then provides a record of service, which is reviewed and approved by a designated individual at the device manufacturer.

Some adjustments may be allowed to be made by operators as part of normal production operations. The allowable adjustments are defined in process specifications or procedures, which are maintained in the work area in the form of an approved chart posted on equipment, as part of the DMR, or as a procedure available to the operator.

820.70(h) MANUFACTURING MATERIAL

The Requirement

820.70(h) Manufacturing material. Where a manufacturing material could reasonably be expected to have an adverse effect on product quality, the manufacturer shall establish and maintain procedures for the use and removal of such manufacturing material to ensure that it is removed or limited to an amount that does not adversely affect the device's quality. The removal or reduction of such manufacturing material shall be documented.

Discussion of the Requirement

Section 820.3(p) defines manufacturing material as "any material or substance used in or used to facilitate the manufacturing process, a concomitant constituent, or a byproduct constituent produced during the manufacturing process, which is present in or on the finished device as a residue or impurity not by design or intent of the manufacturer." Examples of such substances are cleaning agents, mold-release agents, lubricating oils, latex proteins, sterilant residues, and other materials or substances that naturally occur as part of the manufacturing process.

The manufacturer is responsible for evaluating manufacturing materials used during the manufacturing process and for determining the effect of such materials on a device's fitness for use. This requirement applies only when the manufacturing material could potentially have an adverse effect on product.

Under the requirements of section 820.70(h), manufacturers are expected to establish procedures for the use and removal of any manufacturing material and to document the removal or reduction of the material. In documenting the removal process, manufacturers are not required to state how much (i.e., what percentage) of the removal occurred by natural means (e.g., evaporation of isopropyl alcohol) versus how much was removed by a subsequent operation designed to remove residual material that was not removed by natural means. Depending on the manufacturing material and the device, the degree of control required may vary.

The requirement also applies to processing, reprocessing, repair, and rework. All product supplied by third parties must also be evaluated for any manufacturing materials used and must meet the appropriate specification requirements.

Industry Practice

During the development phase of a project, manufacturers customarily identify the manufacturing materials to be used and evaluate the potential adverse effects of the manufacturing materials on product quality. When required, manufacturers document how a material will be used and how the removal or reduction will be performed. The removal or reduction process is commonly documented as part of the DHR.

For product supplied by third parties, allowable manufacturing materials should be documented in the specification requirements, and the supplier is responsible for documenting the use and removal or reduction of such materials as part of the DHR.

820.70(i) AUTOMATED PROCESSES

The Requirement

820.70(i) Automated processes. When computers or automated data processing systems are used as part of production or the quality system, the manufacturer shall validate computer software for its intended use according to an established protocol. All software changes shall be validated before approval and issuance. These validation activities and results shall be documented.

Discussion of the Requirement

The intent of the Quality System regulation is to ensure that all software used in production or the quality system, whether for design, manufacture, distribution, or traceability, is validated for its intended use. Procedures must be established to ensure that validation is properly performed.

The manufacturer has primary responsibility for ensuring that the software is adequate. Validation requirements apply to software developed in-house by the manufacturer, specific software developed by a third party for the manufacturer, and off-the-shelf software. When a manufacturer purchases off-the-shelf software, the manufacturer must ensure that it will perform as intended in its chosen application. When source code and design specifications cannot be obtained, "black box" testing must be performed to confirm that the software meets the user's needs and is suitable for its intended uses.

Manufacturers must evaluate all automated processes, determine the impact of those processes on product safety, performance, and reliability, and determine the extent of validation required. Software programs that control critical areas will require more extensive validation activity and documentation than those that are of lesser risk or subject to subsequent inspection or review.

Procedures must be established defining how the manufacturer will validate software to ensure that the software will consistently perform as intended in its chosen application and that its use will not result in undetected errors. Such validation activity must also address computer hardware.

While FDA does not specifically define how software validation is to be performed, several documents issued by FDA can be used for guidance in establishing a validation program: *Application of the Medical Device GMPs to Computerized Devices and Manufacturing Processes* (November 1990 draft); *Software Development Activities* (July 1987); and *Reviewer Guidance for Computer Controlled Medical Devices Undergoing 510(k) Review** (August 1991).

---

*A draft revision of this guidance document, entitled *ODE Guidance for the Content of Premarket Submissions for Medical Devices*, was made available for comment on September 3, 1996.

Software and software changes must be formally reviewed and approved before implementation. The impact of a change must be assessed to determine its effect on product quality, including its effect on other software modules in the system. A documented system is expected to be followed to control the use of software (application, versions, changes, manuals) and to ensure its validation. Records must be maintained to demonstrate adequate software validation, including validation of software changes.

Additional guidance on validation principles can be found in Chapter 16.

Industry Practice

The use of computers and automated data processing systems for production and quality systems is commonplace in the medical device industry. Examples of process software include

a) test software used in the testing of subassemblies, such as circuit boards and electronic components, or in final acceptance testing of finished devices;

b) software used to implement and support quality system procedures, such as evaluation of materials or product by test and inspection equipment, calibration, control of DMRs, complaint handling, design, and trend analysis;

c) software used to manage data, where information on a manufacturing process or quality system activity is collected and analyzed without operator intervention to control the activity and/or verify the results, and where action is taken on such results; and,

d) manufacturing software used to control various manufacturing processes and equipment, such as wave solder machines, robotics, computerized numerical control (CNC) machines, environmental chambers, sterilization equipment, and sequential assembly processes.

Manufacturers typically establish a policy for the development and validation of process software, identifying the development process, including the determination of specification requirements; outlining the validation process, including test protocols and approval; defining change control requirements; and identifying required documentation. Software validation procedures also commonly address the manufacturer's validation approach for in-house, third-party, and off-the-shelf software, if applicable.

Software Validation Testing. Manufacturers validate process software in several different ways:

a) The software is validated independently of the process that it controls. This approach is typically used for software that resides in a personal computer and controls a piece of equipment through an electronic interface. This approach is also used for quality system software that resides on a personal computer, personal computer network, or mainframe computer. In the case of quality systems, there are generally self-contained programs that do not have external interfaces other than those needed to access a database.

b) The software is validated as part of the process that it controls. This method of validation is applicable when a piece of computer-controlled manufacturing or test equipment is purchased. The computer is built into the equipment and allows the user to select various options from a menu, enter a variety of parameters, print reports, and control the process by means of limited data entry. Examples are automated test equipment (ATE), ionization detection equipment, and circuit-board test fixtures.

c) In some cases, a piece of computer-controlled manufacturing or test equipment contains software that is not obvious or accessible to the user (e.g., computer-controlled environmental chambers for which the user can only set time and temperature within preset limits). In this case, the software itself cannot be validated by the user. When the process is validated through operational qualification and performance qualification, the internal software is also validated by default. As a result, this software is validated during process validation.

Required Documentation. Validation is documented in a protocol that includes at least software/hardware requirements definition, formal test plans, and acceptance criteria. Validating process software is based on first establishing the requirements for the software, which could include a processing sequence, a description of an existing manual operation, or a database structure with accompanying data manipulations.

Manufacturers document software validation test plans and procedures to ensure that all requirements have been correctly implemented. Specific test cases typically include normal as well as abnormal operation and show that known "bad" parts are identified as failures and "good" parts pass. Parameter limits are validated to show that values within and at the limits are acceptable and that values outside the limits are found to be unacceptable. It is routine for each test case to include the expected results. In the case of quality systems, many programs use off-the-shelf spreadsheets of database systems. Manufacturers do not commonly validate these off-the-shelf systems, but they do validate the specific application programs that use these systems.

The results of validation testing must be documented. It is common to express the test results as actual results versus expected results, which are the basis for determining the pass/fail criteria.

Computerized Numerical Control (CNC) Programs. Computerized numerical control programs fall in the category of software that may be validated as part of the process that it controls. However, such programs require special consideration because of the types of processes that they control. The requirements for a CNC program are typically described in the form of a mechanical drawing; the output is usually a machined part. The CNC program can be validated by machining a number of parts and measuring all dimensions according to the drawing used to develop the program. Each dimension (e.g., hole size, cut angle) should be within the limits of tolerance specified on the drawing.

In many cases, the CNC program is downloaded across a network to the specified CNC machine; alternatively, it can be loaded directly into the machine from a disk. Such programs should be validated when first developed and whenever they are changed. However, CNC machine tools tend to wear out and may require periodic adjustment. These adjustments do not normally require validation, but samples from each newly machined lot are commonly measured as a normal quality assurance activity.

In all cases, the validation is documented, including identification of the program and program version, the date of validation, the number of parts measured, and the actual measurements for each dimension.

Purchased Software. Process software is often purchased in one of the following forms: off-the-shelf, "use as is"; off-the-shelf, modified by the manufacturer; custom software developed by a third party for the manufacturer.

For off-the-shelf software, the requirements are established based on the intended use of the software as it relates to the specific application. The requirements established by the manufacturer (user) are not necessarily based on the user's manual that comes with the software. If purchased software is modified by the manufacturer, the validation specifically addresses the modifications as well as the effects of the modifications on the rest of the system.

For custom-developed software, it is typical for a manufacturer to request that the software be developed according to GMP and other FDA requirements. It is best if the user develops the requirements for the software and determines the criteria for validation and acceptance. Ultimately, it is the responsibility of the manufacturer to ensure that custom software meets the user's requirements.

Revalidation. When a manufacturer modifies a process software program for any reason (e.g., to enhance its capabilities or to fix problems), the software change is revalidated before implementation. The nature of the change is documented, and the validation specifically addresses the change as well as the effect of the change on the system. Documentation of the change and the revalidation is maintained and controlled as part of the DMR.

CHAPTER 15. INSPECTION, MEASURING, AND TEST EQUIPMENT (SUBPART G)

820.72 INSPECTION, MEASURING, AND TEST EQUIPMENT

The Requirement

> **820.72 Inspection, measuring, and test equipment.**
>
> **(a) Control of inspection, measuring, and test equipment.** *Each manufacturer shall ensure that all inspection, measuring, and test equipment, including mechanical, automated, or electronic inspection and test equipment, is suitable for its intended purposes and is capable of producing valid results. Each manufacturer shall establish and maintain procedures to ensure that equipment is routinely calibrated, inspected, checked, and maintained. The procedures shall include provisions for handling, preservation, and storage of equipment, so that its accuracy and fitness for use are maintained. These activities shall be documented.*
>
> **(b) Calibration.** *Calibration procedures shall include specific directions and limits for accuracy and precision. When accuracy and precision limits are not met, there shall be provisions for remedial action to reestablish the limits and to evaluate whether there was any adverse effect on the device's quality. These activities shall be documented.*
>
> **(1) Calibration standards.** *Calibration standards used for inspection, measuring, and test equipment shall be traceable to national or international standards. If national or international standards are not practical or available, the manufacturer shall use an independent reproducible standard. If no applicable standard exists, the manufacturer shall establish and maintain an in-house standard.*
>
> **(2) Calibration records.** *The equipment identification, calibration dates, the individual performing each calibration, and the next calibration date shall be documented. These records shall be displayed on or near each piece of equipment or shall be readily available to the personnel using such equipment and to the individuals responsible for calibrating the equipment.*

Discussion of the Requirement

To provide confidence in decisions or actions based on measurement data, proper calibration, storage, and handling controls must be maintained for all measuring and test systems used in the development, production, installation, and servicing of product. Calibration should be performed at least over the range of use of the particular instrument so that the accuracy of the "usable" portion of the instrument is known. All measuring and test equipment must be calibrated and maintained according to written procedures.

Calibration procedures must include accuracy and precision limits and specify the ranges over which the calibrations must be performed. Calibration procedures must specify the remedial action process to be followed if a piece of measurement equipment is found to be out of calibration. Remedial action involves not only an evaluation of the measures required to recalibrate (or, if necessary, replace) the equipment, but also an evaluation of the effects of the out-of-calibration equipment on the quality of any materials, parts, components, packaging, or finished devices produced since the last successful calibration.

Standards used for calibration should be traceable to NIST standards or similar recognized international standards. The standards used must be generally accepted as the prevailing standards. If such standards do not exist, the manufacturer should use an independent, reproducible standard or create and maintain an appropriate, reproducible, in-house standard.

Calibration records must include the actual calibration results, the date of calibration, the signature or other identification of the person who performed the calibration, and the next calibration date. The equipment must also be clearly identified in the calibration records. If the records are not displayed on or near the equipment, they must be readily available to personnel who use the equipment so that the calibration status is readily known and out-of-calibration equipment will not be used.

The necessary accuracy, precision, and resolution required of the measuring and test equipment must be considered and will depend on the required degree of accuracy of the measurements for which the equipment is being used. Calibration procedures also must account for any environmental controls that may be necessary to properly perform the calibration(s). The procedures also should indicate how the equipment should be properly handled and stored after use to ensure that the equipment is properly maintained and protected from adjustments that could invalidate the calibration. Provisions must be in place to ensure that improperly calibrated equipment is not used.

Industry Practice

Manufacturers commonly develop an overall calibration procedure to describe a general calibration policy for measurement equipment. Examples of measurement equipment include gauges, sensors, meters (e.g., voltmeters, pH meters), timers, thermocouples, and software/firmware erasure devices. Typically, separate individual procedures are used to perform the actual calibration of each piece of equipment.

Most manufacturers consider the necessary accuracy, precision, and resolution required for the measuring and test equipment during the establishment of their manufacturing and test procedures. Otherwise, the manufacturer may discover at a later date that the equipment is not suitable (i.e., not accurate or precise enough to provide reliable measurement/test results).

The initial frequency with which measurement and test equipment is calibrated usually is based on the equipment supplier's recommendations. As a manufacturer gains experience with a particular piece of equipment, it may be found necessary to change this frequency.

Accuracy is basically defined as conformance to a traceable standard, and precision is the repeatability of or closeness between measurement results obtained during calibration. Generally, measuring equipment is at least four times, preferably ten times, more accurate than specified tolerances. Traceable standards are typically at least four times, preferably ten times, more accurate than the particular measuring or test equipment being calibrated. The ANSI/ASQC standard, *Calibration Systems*, discusses quantification of calibration errors and provides additional information on determining the degree of uncertainty of a calibration system to ensure that traceable standards are accurate enough for use in a specific calibration program.

Manufacturers commonly define within the general calibration procedure the action to be taken when a calibration exercise results in an out-of-tolerance determination. Manufacturers that evaluate the effects of out-of-calibration results frequently document this evaluation on the calibration records themselves. Many manufacturers perform root-cause investigations to determine why out-of-calibration results are occurring and to prevent them from recurring; this is an important and necessary part of the quality assurance program.

If corrective action is necessary, it is important to determine the cause of the out-of-calibration problem so that it can be prevented in the future. For example, should the frequency of calibration be increased? Should daily or weekly instrument checks be instituted? Is adequate equipment storage available? The results of this analysis may mean that reworking, scrapping, retesting, and/or field corrective action will be necessary.

Some manufacturers are actually plotting quantitative calibration results using percent error versus time to determine any trends in calibration results. This information is used to adjust calibration frequencies accordingly.

Typically, calibration records include the actual calibration results (i.e., the readings before and after calibration) so that, if required, appropriate remedial action can be taken. If calibration results only indicate "in calibration" or "out of calibration and adjustments were made," there will be insufficient information to perform an adequate investigation and determine the appropriate remedial action. In addition, calibration records commonly include or reference other information such as the date of calibration, identification of the person who performed the calibration, and the standards used, so that appropriate remedial action can be taken if required.

Companies generally assign calibration responsibilities to one individual or department. Maintenance of the calibration program, including procedures, documentation, and the physical care of the equipment, are coordinated or directly handled by that individual or department. Calibration functions include indicating the calibration status of each piece of measurement equipment, so that if a processing operation requires the use of a calibrated piece of measurement equipment, its status can readily be determined before use. For this purpose, a calibration sticker can be applied to the equipment, indicating the calibration date, the calibrator, and the due date for the next calibration; or the calibration records can be maintained near the point of use or in an easily accessible location.

Many manufacturers use outside calibration laboratories. Unfortunately, outside calibration laboratories do not always document all calibration results, nor do many of them understand and/or have knowledge of the medical device GMP calibration requirements. To remedy this situation, many manufacturers are performing audits of calibration laboratories when on-site calibrations cannot be performed. Since proper evaluation of calibration laboratories is required under section 820.50, it will be in the manufacturer's interest to ensure that the procedures of outside calibration laboratories comply with GMP requirements and any other established quality criteria.

Some manufacturers have calibration laboratories perform calibration on-site, to the extent possible, so that the calibration laboratory's procedures can be audited during the calibration process. Some calibration laboratories will provide copies of their calibration procedures so that the manufacturer can review them and ensure compliance with GMP requirements.

Many manufacturers use "checks" between normal calibrations to detect any equipment drift before an out-of-calibration condition occurs. For example, standards of known accuracy are used to perform daily checks of certain types of equipment (e.g., scales). These daily checks are recorded on a log sheet. This is good preventive action, since the amount of necessary remedial action is proportional to the amount of time between calibrations. In other words, the sooner a problem is detected, the easier it is to narrow down the affected materials or products and take corrective action.

Regardless of whether calibrations are performed in-house or by calibration laboratories, manufacturers may go to great lengths to prevent equipment from going out-of-tolerance. In addition to the possibility of an out-of tolerance piece of measurement equipment resulting from improper handling and storage, manufacturers have to consider the cost of recalibrating that piece of equipment. For example, a manufacturer may determine that it is necessary to use an appropriate soft cloth to remove hand oils from pin gauges or to use a storage box with soft cloth lining to protect gauges from scratches. These practices may be described in the calibration procedures themselves or in a separate procedure describing the care of the equipment during handling and storage.

CHAPTER 16. PROCESS VALIDATION (SUBPART G)

820.75 PROCESS VALIDATION

The Requirement

820.75 Process validation.

(a) Where the results of a process cannot be fully verified by subsequent inspection and test, the process shall be validated with a high degree of assurance and approved according to established procedures. The validation activities and results, including the date and signature of the individual(s) approving the validation and where appropriate the major equipment validated, shall be documented.

(b) Each manufacturer shall establish and maintain procedures for monitoring and control of process parameters for validated processes to ensure that the specified requirements continue to be met.

(1) Each manufacturer shall ensure that validated processes are performed by qualified individual(s).

(2) For validated processes, the monitoring and control methods and data, the date performed, and, where appropriate, the individual(s) performing the process or the major equipment used shall be documented.

(c) When changes or process deviations occur, the manufacturer shall review and evaluate the process and perform revalidation where appropriate. These activities shall be documented.

Discussion of the Requirement

It is the intent of the Quality System regulation to define the essential elements necessary to ensure that a medical device will consistently meet its predetermined specifications. The FDA's *Medical Device GMP Guidance for FDA Investigators* states that the manufacturer "must establish process controls to insure that the device(s) is not adversely affected by the process and that the process will achieve its intended purpose. Process controls include standards, blueprints, first-piece evaluation, written instructions, operation certification, engineering drawings, inspection, test, etc. as well as *process validation*" (emphasis added).

Section 820.3(z) defines "validation" as a "confirmation by examination and provision of objective evidence that the particular requirements for a specific intended use can be consistently fulfilled." "*Process* validation" is defined in section 820.3(z)(1) as "establishing by objective evidence that a process consistently produces a result or product meeting its predetermined specifications."

Manufacturers are expected to evaluate the processes used to manufacture their devices and determine which "cannot be fully verified by subsequent inspection and test." These processes are subject to the requirements of section 820.75. When a determination not to validate has been made, the rationale supporting the manufacturer's decision should be documented.

In the May 11, 1987, *Federal Register*, FDA published a guidance document, *General Principles of Process Validation*, to help manufacturers understand FDA's policy on validation. The guideline states the key elements that FDA expects to find in process validation:

a) Both the process and the process controls are validated.

b) A written validation protocol specifies the procedures (tests) to be conducted and the data to be collected.

c) The purpose of the data collected is clearly stated.

d) The data reflect facts.

e) The data are collected carefully and accurately.

f) There is a sufficient number of replicate process runs.

g) Reproducibility is demonstrated.

h) There is an accurate measure of variability among successive runs.

i) Test conditions for runs encompass upper and lower processing limits and circumstances, including those within standard operating procedures, which pose the greatest chance of process or product failure as compared to ideal conditions.

j) There is evidence of the suitability of materials.

k) The performance and reliability of equipment and systems are documented.

The following activities are expected to be performed for a validation study:

a) installation and operation qualification for process equipment;
b) software validation, if applicable;
c) process performance qualification;
d) establishment of a system to ensure timely revalidation;
e) documentation of the validation activities and results; and,
f) approval of the validation activities.

While section 820.75(a) applies to the initial validation of a process, section 820.75(b) applies to the performance of a process *after* validation. Documented methods for monitoring and control are required for validated processes. It is expected that manufacturers will assign the performance of validated processes to personnel qualified for those particular activities. The type and frequency of monitoring and control must be determined by the manufacturer based on the process itself and should be evaluated periodically to ensure that specified requirements are still met, especially during revalidation of the process. In addition, production records for validated processes should identify, when appropriate, the process equipment and the individual performing the process.

Although FDA has not officially published guidelines for defining processes that require validation, information has been presented by the agency at numerous national conferences. The following list, which is not intended to be all-inclusive, identifies processes that traditionally have been considered by FDA to require validation:

Test methods	Plastic bonding	Formulations
Welding	Calibration	Software controlled processes
Air systems	Wave/hand soldering	Water systems
Injection molding	Utilities	Extrusion
Sanitization	Dipping	Cleaning
Mixing	Aseptic processing	Lyophilization
Sterilization	Sealing	Filling
Unique filtration		

Rework methods must also be reviewed to determine the need for validation. Rework may adversely affect the safety and effectiveness of the product, and this possibility must be eliminated before a particular method is used. A manufacturer must decide on the need for validation based on knowledge of the product, the process, and the interaction between product and process.

The FDA has identified conditions that would require the associated process activities to be reviewed and evaluated for validation or revalidation:

Stability test failures	Rejects
Reinspection	Retest
Scrap	Troubleshooting
Sorting substandard material	Recalls
Complaints and MDRs	Returns due to quality problems
Excessive warranty/service reports	Failure investigation results
Collection/analysis of samples	

All changes to validated processes also must be reviewed for the need to revalidate. As noted in FDA's *Medical Device GMP Guidance for FDA Investigators*, "all changes to processes must be properly reviewed, validated, documented, and communicated in a timely manner."

Industry Practice

Two types of validation are commonly utilized by device manufacturers, retrospective and prospective. Retrospective validation, as defined in FDA's *General Principles of Process Validation*, is "validation of a process for a product already in distribution based upon accumulated production, testing and control data." Prospective validation is defined as "validation conducted prior to the distribution of either a new product, or product made under a revised manufacturing process, where the revisions may affect the product's characteristics."

In retrospective validation, the expectation is that the adequacy of the process will be demonstrated by examination of accumulated test data on the product and records of the manufacturing procedures used. Retrospective validation is not always acceptable, because the data collected do not lend themselves to analysis for statistical confidence. The accumulated data need to be more than pass/fail results demonstrating lot-to-lot conformance to specifications. This type of validation requires measurement data and the maintenance of records that describe the operating characteristics of the process, such as time, temperature, humidity, and equipment settings.

Prospective validation is usually applied when a product or process is initially released to manufacturing or when there is a major change to the product or process. This type of validation requires all the elements stated previously. Again, the emphasis is on evidence, with a high degree of assurance, of process reproducibility.

Manufacturers use various types of systems to validate processes and to ensure the proper monitoring and control of those processes. An effective program adequately addresses the assignment of responsibilities. Regardless of the size of the manufacturer, it is common for validation activities to be supported by various groups with different specialties, such as engineering design, product operations, and quality assurance personnel. This diversity helps to increase the probability that all relevant information about a particular product and process will be made available.

In addition, the elements described in the following paragraphs are utilized by manufacturers, as appropriate, to ensure adequate validation of processes.

Installation/Operation Qualification: Installation qualification studies are performed to establish confidence that the process equipment and ancillary systems are capable of consistently operating within established limits and tolerances. The equipment is evaluated and tested to verify that it is capable of operating satisfactorily within the operating limits required by the process. Examples of equipment performance characteristics that might be measured include temperature and pressure parameters for injection molding machines; uniformity of speed of mixers; temperature, speed, and pressure of packaging machines; and temperature and pressure of sterilization chambers.

Installation/operation qualification studies include examination of the equipment design; determination of calibration, maintenance, and adjustment requirements; and identification of critical equipment features that could affect the process and product. While it is typical to use the equipment manufacturer's recommendations as an initial basis for assessing equipment design, it is usually not sufficient to rely solely on these recommendations. The device manufacturer may use the equipment differently, for a different purpose, or in different operating ranges and conditions. For a process that has been determined to require validation, each piece of equipment should be assessed in an installation/operation qualification study. Equipment can sometimes be retrospectively qualified. Although some manufacturers argue that installation/operation qualification requirements do not apply to equipment used in established processes, because the equipment was installed perhaps years previously and has been working fine, this is not an acceptable practice.

Installation/operation qualification also commonly includes a review of the pertinent maintenance procedures, repair parts lists, and calibration methods for each piece of equipment.

When possible, installation/operation qualification simulates actual production conditions, including worst-case conditions. Tests and challenges are repeated a sufficient number of times to ensure reliable and meaningful results. Acceptance criteria are defined, and all criteria must be met during the test or challenge. If a failure occurs, an evaluation is performed to identify the cause of the failure. Corrections are made, confirmation test runs performed, and the results documented to provide evidence that the correction was appropriate and solved the problem.

Variability between runs in the installation/operation qualification runs is used to determine the total number of trials selected for the subsequent process performance qualification studies.

Process Performance Qualification: Performance qualification is performed to demonstrate the effectiveness and reproducibility of the process. Performance qualification is conducted by a manufacturer after process specifications have been established and proven by testing or other trial methods and the equipment has been found to be acceptable in the installation/operation qualification studies. Each manufacturing process is qualified and validated separately, as it is not typically acceptable to rely on similarities between products, processes, and equipment without appropriate challenges of each manufacturing process.

During performance qualification, variables that may affect important product quality attributes are challenged. In challenging a process to assess adequacy, a manufacturer challenges conditions that will be probable in the real manufacturing day-to-day environment, including any probable worst-case conditions. The challenges are repeated enough times to ensure meaningful and consistent results. Each manufacturer determines the number of repetitions that is adequate, but this decision is only valid when substantiated by data and statistical rationale.

> NOTE -- Over the years, however, it has become known through FDA statements, notices of observations (FD-483s), establishment inspection reports (EIRs), and warning letters that FDA expects a minimum of three successive, replicate runs during process performance qualification.

Revalidation: Most manufacturers consider revalidation whenever there are changes in the process and/or product. For example, product batch sizes increase or decrease; or changes occur in manufacturing equipment, equipment operating parameters, process location, component manufacturer, methods of formulation, formulas, analytical techniques, packaging, or processes that could affect product effectiveness or product characteristics.

It is common for revalidation concerns to be addressed in QA procedures or the original validation protocol. This system is often integrated with the change control system. When a change is proposed, it is evaluated according to the revalidation procedures. The extent of revalidation will depend upon the nature of the change and how it affects the process and/or the product.

Documentation: Protocols, procedure reports, and the data collected commonly make up the documentation that supports a validation study. A process required to be validated typically is not released for use in routine manufacturing without an approved, documented validation study.

Test data are only considered useful if the methods and results are specific enough to substantiate conclusions. It is insufficient for a manufacturer to assess the process solely on the basis of lot-by-lot conformance to specifications if test results are merely expressed in terms of pass/fail or attribute data. Quantitative, measurable data can be statistically analyzed and a determination made of the variance in data that can be anticipated. Operating characteristics and equipment settings are typically recorded during the validation and made part of the process controls applied to routine manufacturing.

The examples described in the following paragraphs highlight various types of validations and typical approaches used for validation throughout the industry.

Test Methods: The purpose of test method validation is to provide evidence that the method is appropriate for the specification being assessed, that the method is specific and sensitive enough to discriminate a borderline acceptable product from an unacceptable product, and that the test method is accurate, precise, and reliable over repeated applications.

Facility Design: Among the considerations are the following:

a) *Space to operate the process properly.* Adequate space is needed to prevent damage to materials, to clean and maintain equipment properly, and to move materials and product in a manner that will prevent damage and mixups. Parameters to be addressed include the dimensions of the facility and the layout of the equipment, furniture, personnel, materials, power sources, and support systems.

b) *Construction and other materials.* Materials used in facility construction are chosen to prevent environmental and product contamination and to be easily cleaned. Requirements include ceiling material that is nonshedding and nontoxic; wall and floor materials or finishes that are easily cleaned, nonshedding and nontoxic; personnel dress materials that are nonshedding, do not support microbial growth, and can easily be cleaned/sterilized or are disposable; work surfaces that are easily cleaned and/or sanitized, nonporous, and nonshedding.

c) *Support systems.* Support systems such as air conditioning, heating, air filtration (e.g., high-filtration particulate air [HEPA] filters), water (sterile, nonpyrogenic, distilled, treated by reverse osmosis), compressed air, compressed gases, and liquid gases may be needed to create the environment required to meet product and process specifications. Relevant parameters include number of air changes, amount and speed of air flow, temperature, relative humidity, efficiency of cooling, microbial levels in water, number of particulates in air and water, inorganic and organic contaminant levels, and characteristics of prefilters.

d) *Type of manufacturing area.* This specification is determined by the requirements of the product. The required environment might, for example, be a noncontrolled white room or a classified clean room.

e) *Need for monitoring.* Facility monitoring may be necessary to ensure that the specifications approved for the facility design are reliable over time and to provide feedback for preventive maintenance. Among the considerations are preventive maintenance procedures for each system, frequency of monitoring, type of monitoring, calibration of monitoring equipment, and trend analysis of data collected.

Air Systems: Validation of air systems usually includes a review of the system requirements, the installation, and the maintenance history. However, some form of current validation also is performed, such as an examination to verify current installation characteristics and current operating capability.

Some elements to be examined include the chiller systems for the air conditioning systems. Typical parameters examined are power, capacity, capability, and the controls included in the chillers for proper performance and maintenance of the cooling parameters. Other elements of air systems include volume of air, the recirculation of air, air exhaust, air quality, compressor requirements, and controls for proper performance and maintenance.

Water Systems: If the water can contaminate or create an environment for contaminating the product, the installation of the system is typically evaluated as well as any elements of its installation that could contribute to contamination.

A common water treatment system is reverse osmosis. Characteristics of reverse osmosis systems that are commonly evaluated include the source of the water, the capacity of the system to produce and maintain a stated volume, the parts of the system that treat the water, the delivery path controls, and the method of water distribution. The materials of which the water treatment and delivery system are composed also are evaluated to ensure that they meet specifications and that the water will be processed correctly.

Utilities: Validation of power utilities usually involves evaluation of the power fluctuations and power reductions at the source into the manufacturing facility and as it is distributed throughout the facility. Measurements are taken and evaluated with respect to the needs of the processes and support systems within each manufacturing facility and, if applicable, within multiple buildings. Consideration is given to the reliability of the utilities and how any variations will affect process reliability. The worst-case challenge for this type of validation is to evaluate the amount of fluctuation, reduction, or spiking that occurs when the maximum number of systems and equipment are using power at the same time. Power utilities are commonly evaluated and monitored over a period of time to determine normal patterns and to assess whether the utilities will support the needs of the process reliably over time.

Cleaning, Sanitization, Degreasing: When deciding whether to validate a cleaning, sanitizing, or degreasing operation, manufacturers take into account the purpose of the process, considering in the evaluation the product specifications and requirements as well as the needs and requirements of subsequent processes.

Aseptic Processing: Validation of aseptic processing is similar to validation of cleaning and sanitization processes. Issues to be addressed include the quality of the filling and closing environment in terms of minimizing microbial contamination. Among the process elements normally controlled are buildings and facilities, components, containers/closures, production time, laboratory variables, and sterility testing. Validation considerations include air quality and control; facility cleaning; the microbiological quality of components, containers, closures, and the aseptic processing facility; and depyrogenation of containers/closures.

Unique Filtration Processes: The purpose of the filtration aids a manufacturer in determining the intensity of the validation required. Sterile filtration requires the most intense validation and involves use of a microbial challenge. The filter is challenged with the worst-case microbial population and organism, and the challenge is repeated for a sufficient number of trials to ensure reliable performance to meet specifications. The principle used is that if the filtering process can adequately filter the smallest organism at a population 1,000 to 100,000 times that of the normally expected microbial population, the filter can adequately remove organisms found in routine manufacturing. Environmental controls are maintained and monitored to control the microbial population at an acceptable level and to identify changes that could affect the validation.

Filling Operations: Validation of filling operations is primarily concerned with fill volume and contamination of the product. If the product is to be filled sterile, then aseptic processing validation is performed. If the product will be terminally sterilized, then the facility design, environmental monitoring, support systems, and control of materials are validated separately. Pumps used for filling are designed and qualified to prevent contamination. Controls commonly include preventive maintenance and a cleaning, sanitization, and sterilization program to ensure the cleanliness of the pump before each use.

Plastic Bonding: The manufacturer's main focus for this validation is the bond and how it is formed. Examples of parameters associated with various types of bonding include the amount of energy applied, dwell time, dimensions, type of solvent, and amount of solvent. Such parameters are routinely monitored during a bonding process.

Calibration: As recognized national or world standards are typically used for calibration, calibration methods are not routinely validated. When no standard calibration method is available and the manufacturer has to develop one, the new method is qualified and validated.

Wave/Hand Soldering: Typical parameters that can influence wave soldering processes are wave height, the distance of the printed circuit board (PCB) from the wave crest, the speed of the PCB through the equipment, the temperature of various equipment zones, the temperature of the PCB, and the temperature, cleanliness, and level of solder. Whether or not a hand soldering process needs to be validated depends on the use of the soldering. Parameters reviewed include the temperature of the soldering gun, its ability to maintain a stable temperature, the condition of the flux and the solder, and the procedure used to define the process.

Plastic Injection Molding/Extrusion: Many variables can affect the quality of a molded part: barrel temperature; ram pressure; screw speed; the type, temperature, and moisture content of the material; mold temperature; cooling rate; mold design and flow characteristics; cycle time; and the configuration of the part. Extrusion processes operate on principles similar to molding processes, but parts are made by pushing the heated material through a die rather than into a mold.

Dipping Plastic and Rubber: Variables associated with dipping plastic and rubber include the formulation of the material, the batch-to-batch variability of the formulation, environmental temperature and humidity, the time limitations of production, the number of "dips," and whether the dipping operation is manual, automated, or a combination of the two.

Mixing: The principal concern in a mixing process is the homogeneity of the mixture produced by the process. Among the factors that affect mixing are the types of materials being mixed, the characteristics of the materials (e.g., thickness, mixability), the equipment used, the speed of mixing, any sampling of the mixture, and the length of time the material is mixed.

Lyophilization: Among the factors that affect lyophilization processes are the stability of the utilities, the temperature of the cooling water in refrigeration units, the condenser temperature, the vacuum levels, the rate of heat transfer, the sublimation rate, the shelf loading and freezing rate, the frozen product dwell time and temperature, the shelf temperature ramp and soak functions, and product temperature. The parameters that define the quality of the product include phase transition temperature, moisture content, reconstitution rate, product assay, and pH.

Packaging Operations: Considerations involved in the validation of a packaging operation include the purpose of the product being packaged, the function performed by the packaging, and the type of packaging. Examples of packaging parameters include temperature, dwell time, pressure, ultraviolet energy level, and the speed of the conveyor through the ultraviolet tunnel or form, fill, and seal machine. Packages sealed to provide sterile barriers are commonly assessed for seal strength and leakage, primarily at the microbial level.

Sterilization: Various sterilization processes are used in the medical device industry, including dry heat, steam, ethylene oxide, plasma, radiation, and hydrogen peroxide. Factors that influence sterilization processes include the materials used in the product, the orientation of the product within the process, the density of the product and its packaging, humidification of the product, and equipment performance. Some parameters are unique to a particular sterilization process, such as gas concentration in ethylene oxide sterilization and conveyor speed in gamma and electron beam radiation sterilization. Although different parameters may be monitored in different sterilization processes (e.g., vacuum, temperature, and dwell time for gas sterilization; dose, time, and distance from the energy source for radiation sterilization), the purpose of validation is the same. Process performance is monitored, and product samples or biological indicators are tested for sterility.

Formulation Methods: Formulation methods usually address the number of ingredients and the order and manner in which they are added together. Factors influencing the final result include the condition of the ingredients at the time of addition, the order in which the ingredients are added, the condition of the ingredients already added, the time of addition, and any heating and/or cooling needed to achieve the proper formulation.

Software-Controlled Processes: Manufacturers validate software that contributes to the quality of the device, either directly by supporting manufacturing processes or indirectly by supporting quality systems. Such software includes that used in data processing systems that support design, manufacturing, distributing, tracking, or other quality activities. Software programs purchased off-the-shelf are validated for their intended use.

Typically, software purchased with equipment was developed by the equipment manufacturer, and the software code is unknown or inaccessible. This type of software is usually validated using a "black box" approach; that is, the software is exercised for functionality only and is not validated at the code level. Manufacturers evaluate software for proper installation and proper function by designing a set of test conditions and expected inputs to test the software's performance in its environment. Expected inputs include probable process errors.

Validation also is required for software used to support data analysis. The extent or depth of validation of support software depends on the use of the software and on whether the software has been customized by the manufacturer. A common validation approach for off-the-shelf, "used as is" software is to demonstrate that it has been installed correctly and that the functions used produce valid results from the data input.

Software validation is discussed in more detail in Chapter 14.

Manual Processes: Processes performed manually (i.e., processes whose output is primarily controlled by a person's actions) are not validated in the classic sense. Because of the unpredictable sources of variation, these processes can only be qualified. However, to meet the intent of the validation requirements, these processes should be qualified. The philosophy and concept of validation are the same, but the application is different. The intent is still to demonstrate, by objective evidence, that the process is repeatable and that this conclusion can be substantiated with a stated statistical confidence level.

PRODUCT CONTROL

CHAPTER 17. LABELING AND PACKAGING CONTROL (SUBPART K)

820.120 DEVICE LABELING

The Requirement

820.120 Device labeling. Each manufacturer shall establish and maintain procedures to control labeling activities.

(a) Label integrity. Labels shall be printed and applied so as to remian legible and affixed during the customary conditions of processing, storage, handling, distribution, and where appropriate use.

(b) Labeling inspection. Labeling shall not be released for storage or use until a designated individual(s) has examined the labeling for accuracy including, where applicable, the correct expiration date, control number, storage instructions, handling instructions, and any additional processing instructions. The release, including the date and signature of the individual(s) performing the examination, shall be documented in the DHR.

(c) Labeling storage. Each manufacturer shall store labeling in a manner that provides proper identification and is designed to prevent mixups.

(d) Labeling operations. Each manufacturer shall control labeling and packaging operations to prevent labeling mixups. The label and labeling used for each production unit, lot, or batch shall be documented in the DHR.

(e) Control number. Where a control number is required by [section] 820.65, that control number shall be on or shall accompany the device through distribution.

Discussion of the Requirement

As part of the DMR, each manufacturer must develop written specifications for labeling that include requirements for the physical design (e.g., material of construction, dimensions, color, appearance) and content of the labeling. In addition, manufacturers are required to establish written procedures to maintain labeling integrity (legibility and application) and to prevent mixups from occurring during handling, storage, and distribution. The integrity of the label should be demonstrated through qualification under actual processing conditions.

In accordance with written procedures, manufacturers must examine labeling (printed packaging and label material, including containers, lid stock, pouches, bags, instructions) for conformance to specification requirements before it is used. Records of such inspections must be maintained with, or referenced by, the DHR and must include the date and the signature(s) of the individual(s) who performed the examination. When specific information (e.g., expiration date, control number) is printed on the label, that information must be verified before packaging and labeling activities are initiated.

Written control procedures are required when segregation of labels during storage and during packaging and labeling operations must be maintained in order to prevent a labeling mixup. In addition, it is expected that the manufacturer will establish written control procedures for performing inspections of the line, line clearance activities, or label reconciliation activities in the area of the facility in which packaging and labeling will take place to ensure removal of devices and labeling from a previous operation, including any in-process rejects.

Industry Practice

It is common for manufacturers to perform design validation of device labeling under actual conditions of processing, including, for sterile devices, actual sterilization process conditions. Three production runs are usually performed as part of the evaluation, which is detailed in a written protocol describing the labeling specifications and the packaging and labeling process parameters. Design validation of the packaging and labeling under actual conditions may be performed concurrently, under the same validation protocol.

Manufacturers may employ the following control measures to ensure label integrity and prevent mixups:

a) Written procedures describe the method of label printing (e.g., verification of the revision level, removal/destruction of any excess labels from previous operations, use of approved ink and adhesives) and label control (formal change control for label text, construction, color).

b) Written procedures describe the method of label application (manual versus automated application, validated equipment settings).

c) Written procedures describe the sampling plan and method of inspection for examining labeling before release for storage or use. The results of inspections, including the date and the signature(s) of the person(s) who performed the inspections, are documented in the DHR. Any nonconforming labeling is rejected. If automated readers are used, the process is monitored by a designated individual who examines a sample of labels to confirm the results from the automated reader.

d) Adequate facilities are provided, and written procedures describe the requirements, for label identification, spatial segregation, and limited accessibility to prevent label mixups. Generally, labels are stored in a locked or otherwise secure area that is only accessible to persons with authority for material control. Labeling is frequently identified by an item code number assigned to each label type. The item code number may include the revision level of the label. Obsolete labeling is removed from storage areas for approved labeling and is destroyed to prevent mixups.

e) Written procedures describe the control measures taken during labeling and packaging operations to prevent mixups, such as area inspections of the facility, line clearance activities, or label reconciliation activities, to ensure removal of devices and labeling from previous lots and verification of labeling materials against the DMR before use. During the packaging and labeling operation, manufacturers may choose to implement periodic inspections to confirm label integrity and application or to conduct such inspections on the final lot. Also, upon completion of the sterilization process, finished product specifications often require visual inspection of the device to ensure label integrity (legibility and application).

f) Written procedures describe the assignment and application of a control number on the device or its immediate packaging label.

When packaging and labeling is performed by a third party, including a repacker or relabeler, the manufacturer is responsible for ensuring that appropriate and effective written procedures are established at the firm where packaging and labeling operations are performed.

The type and extent of controls that must be applied are determined by the manufacturer based on the design of the packaging process and the likelihood of a label mixup (given historical trends and corrective and preventive actions).

820.130 DEVICE PACKAGING

The Requirement

820.130 Device packaging. Each manufacturer shall ensure that device packaging and shipping containers are designed and constructed to protect the device from alteration or damage during the customary conditions of processing, storage, handling, and distribution.

Discussion of the Requirement

Manufacturers are required to determine design characteristics and specifications of packaging and shipping containers to ensure protection of the device during routine processing, storage, handling, and distribution. The device packaging specifications must be included as part of the DMR and maintained under a formal change control system that requires review and approval of the design and any design changes.

Industry Practice

It is common for manufacturers to perform design validation of device packaging. Package performance is typically evaluated using real-time and/or accelerated test conditions to determine its acceptability under routine, as well as potentially adverse, conditions that may be encountered during processing, storage, and throughout the device's expected shelf life or expiration dating period.

Studies are typically conducted under a formal validation protocol that defines the packaging material specifications, the processing conditions, and the storage conditions to be used during manufacturing. Three production runs are usually performed to determine conformance to the acceptance criteria for packaging design characteristics that are intended to provide protection against damage or contamination. Design characteristics may include

a) package integrity (seal integrity, seal strength, absence of tears, holes or punctures);

b) maintenance of device sterility after sterilization, microbial barrier properties (demonstrated by microbial challenge testing);

c) toxicological properties (absence of leachables or extractables that may contaminate the device); and,

d) the potential effects of exposure of the device and its packaging to adverse environmental conditions (e.g., temperature, humidity, pressure, light).

As part of the design approval, manufacturers may also evaluate the compatibility of the device, the packaging materials, and the packaging process at various stages, including

a) packaging and labeling of the device (where manual or automated methods are employed for placement of the device in the packaging container and for sealing the container, including heat sealing, capping, forming, and so on);

b) sterilization (for terminally sterilized devices, exposures to sterilization process conditions are necessary to evaluate the compatibility of the device, packaging materials, and packaging seals with the selected sterilization conditions and to determine if reprocessing should be allowed when deviations from the sterilization process or packaging and labeling errors occur);

c) transportation between two or more facilities where packaging, sterilization, and/or distribution may take place at different locations using in-process packing or shipping containers that may or may not become a component of the marketed device when it is distributed or which may be reused (device and packaging may both be reusable, as in the case of surgical gowns); and,

d) storage of the packaged and labeled device throughout the expected shelf life or expiration dating period and between significant manufacturing operations (e.g., storage of the device prior to packaging and labeling).

CHAPTER 18. HANDLING, STORAGE, DISTRIBUTION, AND INSTALLATION (SUBPART L)

820.140 HANDLING

The Requirement

820.140 Handling. Each manufacturer shall establish and maintain procedures to ensure that mixups, damage, deterioration, contamination, or other adverse effects to product do not occur during handling.

Discussion of the Requirement

Under this section of the Quality System regulation, each manufacturer is expected to have a documented system that defines device-handling requirements at all stages of manufacture to prevent mixups, damage, deterioration, or other adverse effects. The system should have the ability to identify and segregate quarantined, accepted, and rejected product, using physical, spatial, labeling, or other means to prevent mixups. In addition, the system should take into consideration factors that may cause deterioration of parts, subassemblies, or finished devices and provide for appropriate measures to address these factors to protect the product.

Industry Practice

Most manufacturers have documented handling systems that provide appropriate measures to identify and protect devices at all stages of manufacture, from components through finished product awaiting distribution.

Manufacturers typically separate stages of manufacturing or assembly by assigned work station, work space, or, when appropriate, separate rooms specifically designated for each significant processing step. For some devices, adequate protection may be achieved by the use of totes or bins that move with the product as it is assembled. Other devices may be adequately differentiated during production by careful in-process labeling of materials and the use of discrete identification systems, such as work order numbers or lot numbers. In addition, paperwork that typically accompanies production, such as production travelers or batch record sheets, may provide an additional measure of assurance.

When deemed necessary, due to product specifications or processing requirements, manufacturers utilize environmental controls to protect product from undesirable exposure to excessive temperature or humidity, particulate contamination, and other environmental stresses. In addition, damage or deterioration of parts or product is often addressed by means of packaging controls and/or controls provided by the physical design of the manufacturing facility.

820.150 STORAGE

The Requirement

820.150 Storage.

(a) Each manufacturer shall establish and maintain procedures for the control of storage areas and stock rooms for product to prevent mixups, damage, deterioration, contamination, or other adverse effects pending use or distribution and to ensure that no obsolete, rejected, or deteriorated product is used or distributed. When the quality of product deteriorates over time, it shall be stored in a manner to facilitate proper stock rotation, and its condition shall be assessed as appropriate.

(b) Each manufacturer shall establish and maintain procedures that describe the methods for authorizing receipt from and dispatch to storage areas and stock rooms.

Discussion of the Requirement

Manufacturers must establish systems for storing components, manufacturing materials, subassemblies, finished devices, packaging, and labeling that provide for physical barriers, procedural controls, or both, to preclude mixups, deterioration, or damage to devices during their manufacture, distribution, and installation. Procedures must be established that describe stockroom receipt and issuance practices and ensure that only authorized product is released for use or distribution.

When appropriate, a stock rotation system, such as a "first-in, first-out" (FIFO) system, should be implemented to prevent the use or distribution of product nearing or exceeding a labeled shelf-life limit or expiration date. In addition, such inventory should be periodically checked, inspected, or otherwise assessed to assure that quality requirements are met over time.

Industry Practice

Manufacturers generally establish procedures that describe their product storage practices to prevent mixups and assure that only product meeting its quality requirements is used or distributed.

Identification practices, such as assigning part or lot numbers or indicating "quarantine," "accept," or "reject" product status, are frequently used to differentiate discrete runs of production or batches of raw materials or components. Spatial segregation and/or the use of designated storage bins or locations are also common methods of preventing mixups and/or damage.

Manufacturers frequently restrict access to storage areas to authorized personnel and define specific practices for the movement of stock into and out of assigned areas. These practices generally address the requisition of parts, usage records, the return of unused stock, and required authorizations in order to minimize the possibility of unauthorized product being used or distributed. While consumables may not be assigned part numbers, they may be maintained at an established stock level for general use during production.

For products that have a limited shelf life or that are labeled with a specific expiration date, FIFO stock rotation systems and/or periodic inventory checks are typically employed. Also, when controlled storage environments are necessary to prevent deterioration of the product, manufacturers usually specify, control, and monitor any such requirements and include them in the DMR. These practices allow manufacturers to identify and use inventory before it is rendered unfit for use or to discard any inventory that is unfit for use before it can adversely affect production and the quality attributes of the finished product.

820.160 DISTRIBUTION

The Requirement

820.160 Distribution.

(a) Each manufacturer shall establish and maintain procedures for control and distribution of finished devices to ensure that only those devices approved for release are distributed and that purchase orders are reviewed to ensure that ambiguities and errors are resolved before devices are released for distribution. Where a device's fitness for use or quality deteriorates over time, the procedures shall ensure that expired devices or devices deteriorated beyond acceptable fitness for use are not distributed.

(b) Each manufacturer shall maintain distribution records which include or refer to the location of:

(1) The name and address of the initial consignee;

(2) The identification and quantity of devices shipped;

(3) The date shipped; and

(4) Any control number(s) used.

Discussion of the Requirement

Each manufacturer is expected to have written procedures for the distribution of devices, including the recording of consignee, device identification, lot number, and quantity in each shipment. There must be procedures to ensure that only approved devices are shipped and, in the case of devices that may deteriorate over time, there must be established methods of inspection or other practices that ensure the continued fitness for use of items in approved inventory.

Industry Practice

Manufacturers generally distribute finished devices according to a written procedure that addresses selection of product for shipping, the recording of shipment details on a pick list, invoice or other record, and the retention of hard-copy and/or electronic shipment records.

At some point before a shipment is prepared for distribution, manufacturers conduct a review of the corresponding DHR or production records to ensure that the product meets its quality attributes and that the records themselves are in order. Some manufacturers choose to conduct this review immediately after production so that the product can be moved to an "accept" finished goods storage area and pulled as needed to fill customer orders. Other manufacturers conduct this review as a "toll-gate" or "final check" action as a prerequisite to the product being pulled from inventory.

Regardless of which method is preferred, manufacturers currently employ some method of verifying the acceptability of a finished product prior to distribution. An additional goal of this verification step is to ensure that when deterioration over time is known to occur, expired devices or otherwise deteriorated devices are withheld from distribution.

Distribution records, whether paper or electronic, include the name of the consignee; the part number, lot number or serial number; the quantity shipped; and the date shipped. These records are typically verified for accuracy by a second individual. Aside from business considerations, one goal of the distribution record system is to facilitate an efficient recall should one ever be necessary.

820.170 INSTALLATION

The Requirement

820.170 Installation.

(a) Each manufacturer of a device requiring installation shall establish and maintain adequate installation and inspection instructions, and where appropriate test procedures. Instructions and procedures shall include directions for ensuring proper installation so that the device will perform as intended after installation. The manufacturer shall distribute the instructions and procedures with the device or otherwise make them available to the person(s) installing the device.

(b) The person installing the device shall ensure that the installation, inspection, and any required testing are performed in accordance with the manufacturer's instructions and procedures and shall document the inspection and any test results to demonstrate proper installation.

Discussion of the Requirement

When installation of a device is necessary, the manufacturer must establish adequate instructions and procedures to ensure proper installation and to verify acceptable performance against established specifications. These instructions must be provided or made available to the personnel performing the installation, whether they are the manufacturer's personnel, the customer's personnel, or a third party. The installer must ensure that the installation was done correctly and according to the manufacturer's instructions, and must be able to demonstrate proper installation to FDA through an installation record.

Industry Practice

A manufacturer, the manufacturer's representative, or the customer frequently performs installation according to an installation manual or other form of written instruction, such as a procedure. Installation manuals or procedures may include instructions for installation and operational qualification, testing, inspection, and verification of safety and performance.

Installation checklists are routinely used and retained by both the manufacturer and the customer. Training of customer staff by the manufacturer or the manufacturer's representative is commonly part of the installation process. Many manufacturers treat installation records as an element of the DHR and update them during servicing to reflect and record replacement parts and their lot numbers. Other firms maintain the installation records as part of the service record, cross-referencing to the DHR.

MONITORING AND FEEDBACK

CHAPTER 19. NONCONFORMING PRODUCT (SUBPART I)

820.90 NONCONFORMING PRODUCT

The Requirement

820.90 Nonconforming product.

(a) ***Control of nonconforming product.*** *Each manufacturer shall establish and maintain procedures to control product that does not conform to specified requirements. The procedures shall address the identification, documentation, evaluation, segregation, and disposition of nonconforming product. The evaluation of nonconformance shall include a determination of the need for an investigation and notification of the persons or organizations responsible for the nonconformance. The evaluation and any investigation shall be documented.*

(b) ***Nonconformity review and disposition.*** *(1) Each manufacturer shall establish and maintain procedures that define the responsibility for review and the authority for the disposition of nonconforming product. The procedures shall set forth the review and disposition process. Disposition of nonconforming product shall be documented. Documentation shall include the justification for use of nonconforming product and the signature of the individual(s) authorizing the use.*

(2) Each manufacturer shall establish and maintain procedures for rework, to include retesting and reevaluation of the nonconforming product after rework, to ensure that the product meets its current approved specifications. Rework and reevaluation activities, including a determination of any adverse effect from the rework upon the product, shall be documented in the DHR.

Discussion of the Requirement

Under this part of the Quality System regulation, device manufacturers are expected to have adequate systems and established procedures in place for the identification, control, segregation, evaluation, and disposition of nonconforming product. Each manufacturer's quality system must include controls to ensure that components, manufacturing materials, and finished devices that do not conform to specifications are not inadvertently used or distributed.

The purpose of the required controls is to prevent the use or installation of nonconforming product by ensuring that

a) the authority and responsibility for handling nonconforming components and finished devices are established and communicated;

b) nonconformances are investigated, when appropriate;

c) nonconforming product is held or identified in a manner that will prevent its use; and

d) organizational functions concerned with nonconforming product are properly notified.

When appropriate, nonconforming product must be investigated in accordance with written procedures, and the investigation must be documented. The investigation of nonconformances is an important part of the quality system. The purpose of this activity is to determine the cause and effect of a nonconformance and to prevent its recurrence. The extent of the investigation depends on the particular component or product involved, the degree of complexity, and the suspected or confirmed impact of the nonconformance on product performance or use.

Nonconforming product must be identified and segregated from other similar materials to preclude its inadvertent use until final disposition can be made. Each manufacturer should develop suitable record-keeping procedures to adequately document the product's conformance to specifications.

Reworked or otherwise reprocessed devices and components are to be processed and reinspected in accordance with written procedures to ensure that the reworked device or component meets the original or subsequently modified and approved requirements and that it has no effect on device safety or performance. The manufacturer is required to make a determination as to the effect of reworking on a device, whether there is "repeated" reworking or not.

If a manufacturer decides to use the nonconforming material "as is," this disposition must be documented and an evaluation must be performed to ensure that continued use of the nonconforming material does not compromise the safety and effectiveness of the finished device. The justification for concessions, which FDA requires to be based on scientific evidence and objective decision-making, must be documented. Such concessions should be closely monitored and not become accepted practice.

Industry Practice

Manufacturers use various methods to ensure proper control of nonconforming product. One of the most common is the creation of an MRB or a material review committee (MRC) that is responsible for conferring on the cause and effect of a nonconformance and, in some cases, the feasibility of use of nonconforming product. The members of such groups are identified and authorized, usually by management, to investigate product nonconformances; to establish controls to prevent nonconforming material from being used inadvertently; to evaluate the effect of the possible use of nonconforming product on the functionality of finished devices; to agree on the disposition of nonconforming product; and, to concur on corrective action, as appropriate.

In smaller companies, MRB actions are usually agreed upon by one or more members of the management team or others who are aware of the impact of using the material on the finished device and who are empowered to make the technical decisions.

Regardless of company size, written procedures are employed to characterize the practice used and to designate the responsible individuals with authority to make final decisions. The procedures typically include methods of identifying the product(s) involved; identification of those responsible for making the disposition decision; a written rationale or justification for the disposition decision; and the signatures of those approving the disposition.

These procedures typically include a form for identifying the material, the nature of the problem, those responsible for investigation and follow-up, the proposed disposition, and the corrective action to be taken. One or more approval signatures are typically required for the form or report, which then becomes part of the DHR for the material in question and/or the DHR for the finished device.

Standard dispositions of nonconforming product include

   a) accept-as-is;
   b) accept, with rework or other reprocessing;
   c) reject or scrap;
   d) downgrade for use in other applications; and,
   e) return to supplier.

"Accept-as-is" disposition of nonconforming product is documented with written justification and with approvals by those authorized to release the material.

The procedures also may include the requirement that before a disposition action is taken which directly involves a component supplier or the finished-device purchaser, there should be additional concession approvals by those parties. These approval records are maintained as part of the DHR.

To preclude their unauthorized use until suitable disposition is made, nonconforming materials are usually identified and segregated from other products in a controlled area. Ideally, the material should be tagged and removed to a restricted or quarantined area pending disposition. When nonconformances can be corrected or reworked in a timely manner, the product is not necessarily moved, provided that it is properly identified.

In addition, manufacturers routinely have suitable rework procedures in place to address nonconforming product destined for rework or repair. Reworked product is reevaluated and/or retested to ensure that it meets its original specifications. The results of reworking and reevaluation are then recorded in the DHR.

Information on nonconforming product, its disposition, and any necessary corrective action is typically communicated, although not always in a formal fashion, to the various affected organizational units responsible for the nonconformance. The FDA is now requiring that if a particular person or organization is responsible for a nonconformance, that individual or organization should be notified to ensure that future nonconformances are prevented. While the methods used for this communication will depend on the nature of the nonconformance, it should be done in a timely manner to preclude the specific recurrence. It may be practical for personnel to officially acknowledge receipt of this information in order to provide evidence of compliance with the regulation.

CHAPTER 20. CORRECTIVE AND PREVENTIVE ACTION (SUBPART J)

820.100 CORRECTIVE AND PREVENTIVE ACTION

The Requirement

820.100 Corrective and preventive action.

(a) Each manufacturer shall establish and maintain procedures for implementing corrective and preventive action. The procedures shall include requirements for:

(1) Analyzing processes, work operations, concessions, quality audit reports, quality records, service records, complaints, returned product, and other sources of quality data to identify existing and potential causes of nonconforming product, or other quality problems. Appropriate statistical methodology shall be employed where necessary to detect recurring quality problems;

(2) Investigating the cause of nonconformities relating to product, processes, and the quality system;

(3) Identifying the action(s) needed to correct and prevent recurrence of nonconforming product and other quality problems;

(4) Verifying or validating the corrective and preventive action to ensure that such action is effective and does not adversely affect the finished device;

(5) Implementing and recording changes in methods and procedures needed to correct and prevent identified quality problems;

(6) Ensuring that information related to quality problems or nonconforming product is disseminated to those directly responsible for assuring the quality of such product or the prevention of such problems; and

(7) Submitting relevant information on identified quality problems, as well as corrective and preventive actions, for management review.

(b) All activities required under this section, and their results, shall be documented.

Discussion of the Requirement

This section requires that each manufacturer establish procedures and controls for implementing corrective and preventive action. Manufacturers are expected to analyze those processes related to the production, distribution, and servicing of a product, including customer complaints. Corrective and preventive action may also apply to a manufacturer's design control program, particularly with respect to problems encountered during design reviews, product validation or verification, and process validation. In addition, the quality system must provide for control and action to be taken for both devices distributed and not yet distributed.

Procedures must include or refer to the statistical methodology that employees should use to identify recurring problems. Decisions based on analysis of data will play a key role in the quality improvement effort. Success requires application of the correct analytical tools.

The procedures must clearly define the criteria to be followed to determine what information is relevant to the action taken (or not taken) and why. The FDA has emphasized that it is management's responsibility to ensure that all nonconformances are handled appropriately. An important part of corrective and preventive action is the investigation of a problem in order to identify the action needed to eliminate the cause or source of the problem. An effective investigation will help prevent a potential problem from occurring in the first place or an existing problem from recurring.

The manufacturer must ensure that actions taken to eliminate or minimize the causes of actual or potential nonconformances are appropriate for the magnitude of the problem and for the risks encountered. While the regulation cannot dictate the degree of action to be taken, FDA does expect manufacturers to develop procedures for assessing risk, for the actions to be taken for different levels of risk, and for correcting problems and preventing them from recurring.

Verification or validation of the solution is a vital step in the corrective and preventive action process. After implementation, data should be collected and analyzed to ensure that the action taken was effective and does not adversely affect the product or process in question. Follow-up activity closes the loop on the corrective and preventive action process.

Similarly to the requirement of section 820.90(a), procedures for corrective and preventive action must ensure that proper organizational functions are notified of information related to nonconforming product or quality problems. In addition, relevant information on actions taken must be submitted to management for review in accordance with systems established to meet the requirements of section 820.20(c).

Corrective and preventive action activities and results must be documented. It is important to note that FDA has the authority to review records pertaining to corrective and preventive action. These records are not protected under the regulation in the same manner as internal audit and management review records.

Industry Practice

The Quality System regulation states that the procedures include provisions for analyzing processes, work operations, quality reports and records, service reports, concessions, customer complaints, returned products, management reviews, and other sources of quality data in order to detect existing and potential quality problems. Quality problems might result from

a) improper design;
b) inadequate or nonexistent component or product specifications;
c) failures of or problems with purchased materials;
d) inadequate manufacturing instructions, processes, tools, or equipment;
e) improper facilities or equipment for the storage or handling of materials or products;
f) poor scheduling;

g) inadequate training or lack of training;

h) inadequate or improper working conditions; and/or,

i) inadequate resources.

Regardless of regulatory requirements, managers of successful companies strive to meet their customers' expectations and work on methods for continuous improvement. This is often accomplished by developing a comprehensive, closed-loop corrective and preventive action system that spans the entire organization.

These programs can vary from very broad systems suitable for large diversified organizations to simple systems for small organizations housed in a single location. Regardless of the degree of complexity of a manufacturer's program, the following elements are typically found in an effective system:

a) the organization of people that puts the closed-loop process into practice, including the way that responsibility for managing the system is distributed within the organization;

b) the closed-loop process itself, which is composed of sequential activities that identify, correct, or eliminate existing or potential problems; and,

c) the tools for managing the closed-loop system, which include the written procedures and work instructions used to define the closed-loop process, as well as some form of information system for managing the information associated with corrective and preventive action.

There are many ways of designing and implementing an effective corrective and preventive action program. In one approach, the closed-loop process consists of the following stages:

a) *Documenting the Problem.* This stage has two principle steps: (a) identifying and describing the problem, and (b) assigning a control number for tracking action items.

b) *Establishing a Priority Level and Correcting the Defect.* When a problem is discovered, someone first needs to determine its urgency and importance, which generally depend on the risk associated with the problem. If the problem affects components or finished devices, the next step is to segregate the defective items. A recall may be necessary if the products have already been distributed.

c) *Determining Whether the Problem Requires Action.* Not all problems require action. Simple quality or assembly problems may, for example, be deferred for higher priority items.

d) *Analyzing the Data and Developing an Action Plan.* When action is in order, the root cause of the problem needs to be identified. For complex problems, it may be necessary to develop an action plan and assign responsibility for carrying out various pieces of the plan.

e) *Identifying, Implementing, and Validating the Appropriate Solution.* Analysis of the data may lead to more than one viable solution. The appropriate solution is then selected and implemented. Implementation may require a change order and may have a broad impact on the organization. The solution can be verified, but it may not be possible to fully validate it until the change is implemented in a production environment.

f) *Escalating the Action.* It may be necessary to escalate a corrective or preventive action. Not all action plans proceed as anticipated, and management intervention may be required.

g) *Documentation and Follow-Up Monitoring.* Documentation and follow-up monitoring are the final activities in the corrective and preventive action process. The activities and action are documented, along with any important decisions about the action taken. The action is also monitored to ensure that it was effective and did not adversely affect the finished device. If additional problems are discovered, the process starts over.

CHAPTER 21. COMPLAINT FILES (SUBPART M)

820.198 COMPLAINT FILES

820.198(a)

The Requirement

820.198 *Complaint files.*

(a) Each manufacturer shall maintain complaint files. Each manufacturer shall establish and maintain procedures for receiving, reviewing, and evaluating complaints by a formally designated unit. Such procedures shall ensure that:

(1) All complaints are processed in a uniform and timely manner;

(2) Oral complaints are documented upon receipt; and

(3) Complaints are evaluated to determine whether the complaint represents an event which is required to be reported to FDA under part 803 or 804 of this chapter, Medical Device Reporting.

Discussion of the Requirement

This section of the regulation requires a manufacturer to establish and maintain complaint files, as well as a written procedure for processing complaints. The complaint-handling procedure must provide for the processing of all complaints in a uniform and timely manner, for documentation of oral complaints, and for evaluation of complaints for MDR reportable events under the requirements of 21 CFR 803.

Section 820.3(b) of the regulation defines a "complaint" as "any written, electronic, or oral communication that alleges deficiencies related to the identity, quality, durability, reliability, safety, effectiveness, or performance of a device after it is released for distribution." Based on this definition and the requirements of section 820.198, a report need not be confirmed by a manufacturer in order to be considered a complaint. The FDA expects manufacturers to classify all information that relates to the inadequate performance of a device as a possible complaint. This position has been maintained to ensure that manufacturers consider all sources of alleged device defect information and take appropriate action when problems are found.

The FDA has stated that one group, unit, or individual must be made responsible for coordinating all complaint-handling functions, regardless of how large a manufacturer is, the number of facilities or divisions, the extent of the manufacturer's product lines, or the number of different complaint-handling units within the organization. The intent is to ensure uniformity in the application of the manufacturer's complaint procedure(s). Responsibility may, however, be delegated to appropriate functional units within a company for various aspects of complaint handling, including complaint investigations.

If a manufacturer provides maintenance, service, or repairs for its devices, there must be an adequate system in place to screen requests for repair and service to ensure that any reports representing complaints are handled through the complaint-handling system. In addition, service and repair records must be reviewed for MDR reportable events. Any such reports must automatically be processed as complaints.

Appropriate statistical methods must be used, when necessary, to analyze repair and service quality data to identify potential problems with design, specific components, or premature failures. If trends occur, investigation and appropriate corrective action, when necessary, are required. For those problems determined to be potential hazards to safety, immediate action through an appropriate system is required.

Industry Practice

Most manufacturers have a formal complaint-handling procedure and a documentation system for recording complaints and complaint follow-up. Manufacturers typically focus first on satisfying customer needs and concurrently, or secondarily, on determining whether a quality problem exists, the source of the problem, and the appropriate corrective action.

The manner in which manufacturers handle complaints varies considerably. Small companies often direct all complaints to a single individual or department, while large companies with multiple facilities often designate one functional unit within each facility to coordinate all complaint-handling activities. Manufacturers that also service their devices frequently direct service calls or calls requesting technical information to a different functional unit than the group that handles complaints.

The challenge manufacturers face is to ensure that all information which may represent a "complaint," as defined in the regulation and company procedures, is properly directed and handled, regardless of whether the information comes from customers external or internal to the manufacturer. Good written procedures and extensive training of personnel help to ensure proper complaint handling.

Manufacturers may record complaints manually or enter the information into a computer database. The advantage of using a computer for complaint handling is that most databases can be configured to provide trending information readily. If complaints are not directly input into a computer system, a mechanism is needed to ensure that all complaint information is properly registered and transcribed.

Most companies' written complaint-handling procedures cover all the elements identified in the regulations. An effective documented procedure covers

  a) assignment of responsibility for complaint handling;

  b) the process for defining, recording, evaluating, investigating, and processing complaints;

  c) instructions for obtaining and documenting complaint information, including that pertaining to returned devices;

d) corrective actions;

e) segregation and disposition or reprocessing (including decontamination) of customer returns;

f) the records to be maintained, where customer correspondence and other records are to be filed, and record retention time;

g) complaint closure requirements, including time periods; and,

h) statistical analysis or trending requirements.

The formally designated unit usually has responsibility for tracking complaints to ensure that they are handled in a timely fashion and that appropriate information is provided. The complaint-handling procedure may contain or refer to a separate procedure for screening repair and service requests as complaints, as well for evaluating complaints and requests for repair and service as MDRs.

820.198(b) and 820.198(c)

The Requirement

820.198(b) Each manufacturer shall review and evaluate all complaints to determine whether an investigation is necessary. When no investigation is made, the manufacturer shall maintain a record that includes the reason no investigation was made and the name of the individual responsible for the decision not to investigate.

820.198(c) Any complaint involving the possible failure of a device, labeling, or packaging to meet any of its specifications shall be reviewed, evaluated, and investigated, unless such investigation has already been performed for a similar complaint and another investigation is not necessary.

Discussion of the Requirement

Manufacturers are required to ensure that all complaints are evaluated to determine whether an investigation is needed. Duplicative investigations are not necessary, provided that the manufacturer can demonstrate that the same type of failure or nonconformity has already been investigated. If no investigation is performed, the reason must be documented and signed by the individual who made the decision not to investigate. Unless a similar complaint has already been investigated, a manufacturer is required to conduct an investigation if the device, its labeling, or its packaging may have failed to meet specification.

Industry Practice

As part of their complaint-handling procedures and records, many manufacturers have a step requiring a designated individual to determine whether an investigation is required and, if not, to document the reason. The responsibility for determining whether a complaint investigation is required is usually assigned to an individual with a thorough understanding of the device and an appreciation of the importance of complaint information to a manufacturer's quality system and quality improvement program. The decision-making process is often documented by means of a standardized checklist or decision tree.

The FDA believes that some type of investigation is appropriate for most complaints in order to determine whether the complaint can be confirmed. In addition, as manufacturers implement comprehensive quality systems to make continuous improvements in product quality, they find that thorough investigation of device problems yields useful information.

Such investigation may involve a review of records (e.g., complaint files, DHRs, or other quality system records) to determine if deviations occurred in the manufacturing process or if similar failures have occurred with the product line in question or related product lines. Failure investigation may also involve testing of devices, auditing of suppliers, or other actions appropriate to identify the root cause of a problem.

Most manufacturers typically do not conduct a complaint investigation when they have already identified the problem based upon an earlier complaint or when the complaint is a well known phenomenon unrelated to product quality or performance.

820.198(d)

The Requirement

820.198(d) *Any complaint that represents an event which must be reported to FDA under part 803 or 804 of this chapter shall be promptly reviewed, evaluated, and investigated by a designated individual(s) and shall be maintained in a separate portion of the complaint files or otherwise clearly identified. In addition to the information required by 820.198(e), records of investigation under this paragraph shall include a determination of:*
> *(1) Whether the device failed to meet specifications;*
> *(2) Whether the device was being used for treatment or diagnosis; and*
> *(3) The relationship, if any, of the device to the reported incident or adverse event.*

Discussion of the Requirement

The Quality System regulation clearly mandates that any complaint received by a manufacturer which must be reported to FDA under part 803 or 804 must be immediately processed through the complaint-handling system. The manufacturer is required to conduct an investigation of any such report. These complaints must either be maintained separately in the complaint file or clearly identified as incidents relating to death, injury, or hazards to health.

While FDA expects a manufacturer to make a serious effort to gather information on all complaints, any investigations under this part must contain a determination as to whether the device actually failed, whether the device in question was being used to treat or diagnose a patient, and whether there was any relationship between the device and the reported incident.

Industry Practice

Special provisions to ensure adequate documentation for complaints pertaining to reportable events are common in complaint-handling and MDR reporting procedures. Manufacturers take complaints of this nature very seriously, not only because it is an FDA requirement, but also because there may be serious legal implications.

It is not unusual, however, for a manufacturer to do an inadequate job of documenting the findings in a way that an FDA investigator will understand. Many manufacturers have found that standardizing the process by utilizing checklists and decision trees for all complaints ensures that the necessary information is captured for reports pertaining to death, serious injury, or hazards to safety.

For a number of manufacturers, because of the patient population for whom the device is intended, reports of deaths or serious injuries are not uncommon. For example, manufacturers of implantable defibrillators, anesthesia equipment, apnea monitors, and heart valves receive numerous reports of patient deaths. For companies that manufacture these types of devices, it is important for the manufacturer to determine whether the device caused or contributed to a problem or it was unassociated with the death or injury.

Although an option in the regulation, few manufacturers physically segregate reports of this nature from other complaints. These events are typically identified with unique file numbers, recorded on paper of a different color, or flagged in the computer database.

820.198(e)

The Requirement

820.198(e) When an investigation is made under this section, a record of the investigation shall be maintained by the formally designated unit identified in paragraph (a) of this section. The record of investigation shall include:
   (1) The name of the device;
   (2) The date the complaint was received;
   (3) Any device identification(s) and control number(s) used;
   (4) The name, address, and phone number of the complainant;
   (5) The nature and details of the complaint;
   (6) The dates and results of the investigation;
   (7) Any corrective action taken; and
   (8) Any reply to the complainant.

Discussion of the Requirement

The requirements under this section mandate that a written record be kept of any complaint investigation. The written record of the investigation must be maintained by the formally designated unit with responsibility for complaint files. The specific items required are clearly identified in section 820.198(e). These items include the information that must be collected regarding the complainant and the incident, as well as the details of the investigation and the corrective action taken.

Industry Practice

Many manufacturers try to obtain detailed information about customer complaints so that an investigation can be performed and the problem, if any, identified and corrected. However, the extent to which a manufacturer tries to obtain information about a complaint may be related to the seriousness of the complaint with respect to potential health hazards. Likewise, if a reported problem is one that a manufacturer believes to be well recognized and understood, the amount of inquiry may be more limited than if the problem is a new one.

Incident-Specific Information, Including Device Information. It is often difficult for a manufacturer to obtain complete information from customers, even on details or specifics related to the alleged incident and device in question. Likewise, a manufacturer may simply accept the complaint information provided by the complainant and not ask sufficient additional questions to enable the manufacturer to understand the complaint, make an adequate investigation, or take an appropriate corrective action. The GMP requirements make it clear that manufacturers should either obtain the specified information or document their efforts and their inability to do so.

Investigation Results, Including Corrective Actions. Even when detailed information is available, it is sometimes difficult for a manufacturer to duplicate a reported incident or identify a single cause (or causes) of a particular problem during the investigation. Because FDA implies that the cause of any problem needs to be identified and appropriate corrective action implemented, manufacturers should expend additional efforts in these areas. The results of a manufacturer's investigation typically include the dates of the investigation, the details of the complaint, the details of the investigation, and a description of the corrective action taken.

Reply to the Complainant. Not all manufacturers reply to the complainant. When a reply is made, the method of response varies greatly from manufacturer to manufacturer. For some, a simple verbal communication by telephone or during a visit from the sales representative is typical. Others believe that the response customers find most appropriate is simply to replace problem devices, that customers may not have a real interest in the source or correction of the problem. Some manufacturers not only reply but also provide the results of the investigation and an explanation of any corrective actions taken as a result of the report.

820.198(f) and 820.198(g)

The Requirement

820.198(f) When the manufacturer's formally designated complaint unit is located at a site separate from the manufacturing establishment, the investigated complaint(s) and the record(s) of investigation shall be reasonably accessible to the manufacturing establishment.

820.198(g) If a manufacturer's formally designated complaint unit is located outside of the United States, records required by this section shall be reasonably accessible in the United States at either:

(1) A location in the United States where the manufacturer's records are regularly kept; or

(2) The location of the initial distributor.

Discussion of the Requirement

Complaint files, including records of investigations, must be maintained by the formally designated complaint unit and must be reasonably accessible to the actual manufacturing site (e.g., by means of duplicate paper files or a shared database), when these locations are not the same. The objective of this requirement is to ensure that complaints are reviewed by the actual manufacturing facility so that quality problems can be identified in a timely fashion and appropriate corrective action taken. In addition, FDA must have access to these records in the United States.

Industry Practice

Manufacturers whose complaint-handling functions are at sites separate from the actual manufacturing establishment typically have systems to ensure that copies of complaints associated with the manufacturing process are sent to the actual manufacturer. This applies not only to the corporate headquarters of large companies with multiple facilities, but also to companies that subcontract the manufacture of their finished devices.

Although not an effective or efficient practice, companies with complaint-handling units at facilities remote from the manufacturing site often only notify the manufacturing site after a complaint has been processed and closed. While this practice allows the intent of the Quality System regulation to be met, since the complaint and investigation files are maintained at both locations, little value is added to the investigation of a potential problem. The manufacturing site does not have the opportunity to provide input into decisions, and the complaint-handling unit may be making determinations about whether a particular complaint potentially represents a manufacturing error or deviation and whether an investigation is or is not required.

An effective system requires input from the actual manufacturer during the investigation process, when appropriate, allowing for quick response in the case of an actual manufacturing problem, as well as insight into the potential cause or causes of an alleged product incident report.

Many foreign manufacturers with U.S. importers and distributors permit their U.S. representatives to collect complaint information and forward it to the foreign manufacturer for investigation and resolution. Some foreign manufacturers ask that information be forwarded only for those complaints associated with the design or manufacture of the device. Often, although in violation of the GMP requirements, no information or incomplete information on the disposition of complaints is returned to the U.S. facility.

The Quality System regulation requires that a duplicate of any complaint and the results of the complaint investigation be kept in the United States, at a location readily accessible to FDA. Manufacturers comply with this requirement by sending or faxing written copies of complaints to their U.S. importers, distributors, or representatives, by electronic transfer, or by sharing records.

CHAPTER 22. SERVICING (SUBPART N)

820.200 SERVICING

The Requirement

820.200 Servicing.

(a) Where servicing is a specified requirement, each manufacturer shall establish and maintain instructions and procedures for performing and verifying that the servicing meets the specified requirements.

(b) Each manufacturer shall analyze service reports with appropriate statistical methodology in accordance with [section] 820.100.

(c) Each manufacturer who receives a service report that represents an event which must be reported to FDA under part 803 or 804 of this chapter shall automatically consider the report a complaint and shall process it in accordance with the requirements of [section] 820.198.

(d) Service reports shall be documented and shall include:

(1) The name of the device serviced;

(2) Any device identification(s) and control number(s) used;

(3) The date of service;

(4) The individual(s) servicing the device;

(5) The service performed; and

(6) The test and inspection data.

Discussion of the Requirement

This section applies only to original device manufacturers who service devices and to remanufacturers. Health care facilities that service their own devices and independent third-party servicers are not subject to section 820.200.

Section 820.200 requires manufacturers to establish and implement servicing quality systems that meet all applicable requirements of the regulation. The quality system must ensure that

   a) components used for repair are acceptable for their intended use;

   b) written inspection and test procedures are established;

   c) measurement equipment is properly calibrated and maintained;

   d) serviced devices will perform as intended after servicing;

   e) criteria are established for determining when a service event is an MDR reportable event;

   f) all service events are screened against MDR reporting criteria;

   g) service reports are analyzed using "appropriate statistical methodology";

h) trends are acted upon under the requirements of section 820.100;

i) individuals performing servicing have the appropriate documented training; and,

j) records containing the quantitative inspection/test results and the information required by section 820.200(d) are maintained.

Industry Practice

Some U.S. device manufacturers are ISO certified or in the process of obtaining ISO certification; and many of the GMP requirements for servicing are already in place. Other manufacturers, as a result of prior FDA inspections and ensuing 483s and warning letters, comply with portions of the requirement by maintaining records of service reports and by having servicing procedures that include provisions for determining whether a service report triggers MDR requirements.

Still other manufacturers operate field service activities totally independently of their quality system. Consequently, device problems corrected in the field often are not accurately recorded, or recorded at all, by the manufacturer's quality system, with the result that corrective and preventive action is not implemented and similar problems may recur.

An effective servicing quality system includes provisions to ensure that service records are evaluated to determine if the request must be considered an MDR or a complaint and subject to an investigation. The regulation requires that all service reports classified as MDRs be processed through the manufacturer's complaint-handling system.

The servicing program also may address the following activities:

a) clarification of servicing responsibilities;
b) planning of service activities;
c) validation of special tools or equipment used for repairing and servicing devices;
d) control of measuring and test equipment;
e) control of documentation;
f) training of service personnel; and,
g) feedback and monitoring of service reports and information.

Manufacturers may include servicing activities within other systems and procedures in their quality programs or generate separate systems to handle service activities. Other quality system requirements affected by servicing activities include training; quality audits; purchasing and component controls; inspection and testing; control of inspection, measuring, and test equipment; nonconforming product; corrective and preventive action; documentation controls; and records.

A problem faced by many manufacturers is the failure of field service personnel to accurately report product problems or to provide enough information for a comprehensive failure investigation. This problem can be corrected to some degree by properly training field service personnel in the recognition of product problems that should be reported and in information gathering.

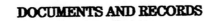

DOCUMENTS AND RECORDS

CHAPTER 23. DOCUMENT CONTROLS (SUBPART D)

820.40 DOCUMENT CONTROLS

The Requirement

820.40 Document controls. *Each manufacturer shall establish and maintain procedures to control all documents that are required by this part. The procedures shall provide for the following:*

*(a) **Document approval and distribution.** Each manufacturer shall designate an individual(s) to review for adequacy and approve prior to issuance all documents established to meet the requirements of this part. The approval, including the date and signature of the individual(s) approving the document, shall be documented. Documents established to meet the requirements of this part shall be available at all locations for which they are designated, used, or otherwise necessary, and all obsolete documents shall be promptly removed from all points of use or otherwise prevented from unintended use.*

*(b) **Document changes.** Changes to documents shall be reviewed and approved by an individual(s) in the same function or organization that performed the original review and approval, unless specifically designated otherwise. Approved changes shall be communicated to the appropriate personnel in a timely manner. Each manufacturer shall maintain records of changes to documents. Change records shall include a description of the change, identification of the affected documents, the signature of the approving individual(s), the approval date, and when the change becomes effective.*

Discussion of the Requirement

Under the general requirements of this section, a manufacturer is expected to establish and maintain, before start-up of production, a documented system to develop, identify, distribute, change, and control all product, process, and quality assurance documentation required by the Quality System regulation and the manufacturer's operation.

The system must encompass all new documents as well as any changes to existing documents. It must ensure that the accuracy and use of documents are controlled, that obsolete documents are removed or prevented from being used, and that all documentation is adequate for its intended use or purpose.

A manufacturer's written procedures must provide methods for

    a) document development, review, and approval to ensure that documents are accurate and meet the requirements of the regulation;

    b) distribution and maintenance to ensure that documents are made available at locations where they are used and to personnel who require them;

c) preparation, review, approval, and qualification of revisions;

d) timely implementation and notification of changes;

e) archiving records of change;

f) retrieval of obsolete or superseded documents to ensure that only the current and approved version is used; and,

g) verification of document distribution and retrieval.

In addition, it is required that those individuals or functions that originally approved a document must review any changes and the effects of such changes on the document, system, and product. However, manufacturers are allowed to specifically designate individuals who did not perform the original review to review and approve changes. In these instances, the manufacturer must determine which individuals or functions are best suited to perform the review and approval.

Requirements for validating changes to specifications, methods, or procedures are addressed in sections 820.30(i), "Design changes," and 820.70(b), "Production and process changes."

Industry Practice

The numerous systems and methods of document control and configuration management used by the medical device industry illustrate that no one documentation control system works for all manufacturers. Systems range from completely manual systems with all paper copies to electronic and paperless systems. Most manufacturers implement a system that is a combination of paper and electronic documentation control.

In one manner or another, document controls affect all aspects of a manufacturer's operation and activities, including design, purchasing, production, testing and inspection, quality assurance, installation, and service. Also encompassed are materials, product, and equipment, such as raw materials, components, software, labeling and packaging, manufacturing materials, finished devices, production equipment and/or tools, measuring equipment and tools, and workmanship standards.

Controlled documents may include, but are not limited to, blueprints, drawings, SOPs, specifications, inspection instructions, test methods, DMRs, forms, and labeling, including labels for in-process and final product. Certain quality system documents and records may also be controlled, such as inspection and test reports, qualification and validation protocols and reports, and audit reports. Both "masters" and "copies" are controlled through the document control system. "Masters" refer to original documents, which are created, approved, changed, and archived, while "copies" are the actual documents circulated and distributed for use.

It is common practice for manufacturers to centralize and assign document control functions to a single individual or department, generally within either the quality assurance department or the engineering department. When the function is centralized, the system typically allows some degree of flexibility by providing for various levels of review and approval of different types of documents and document changes (e.g., administrative changes versus the release of a new document; release of a manufacturing procedure versus release of a product specification). Multiple, noncentralized systems have built-in flexibility, but many manufacturers have found such systems to be more difficult to maintain and control.

Manufacturers commonly describe the document control function in a written procedure in conjunction with one or more forms or checklists, which are often identified as Engineering/Document Change Requests (ECRs/DCRs), Engineering/Document Change Orders (ECOs/DCOs), or Engineering/Document Change Notices (ECNs/DCNs). Such forms capture the reasons for each document and/or change, as well as identify the specific change. They also typically address evaluation of the change; validation, training, and regulatory considerations; distribution and implementation issues; revision level; effectivity; and, disposition of any affected materials.

The mechanics of the document control process typically encompass the following elements:

a) The need for the document, especially revisions to existing documents, is justified.

b) The new document or change to be implemented is identified, as well as the devices, components, subassemblies, labeling, software, processes, and/or procedures that are affected. It is also necessary to identify any primary or secondary document sources, including instruction manuals and labels, that may require review and updating.

c) The new document or document change is evaluated. Factors commonly taken into consideration include regulatory status (e.g., submission requirements or product licensing information), design requirements, and validation requirements. The impact of the new or revised document on other products, documents, or systems is also commonly reviewed. Equally important, although often overlooked, is a financial evaluation of the new document or change.

d) The revision level is identified. A common practice among manufacturers is to use a numeric revision-level system for engineering (preproduction) documents and an alphabetical revision-level system for production documents.

e) The effectivity of the change is assigned by means of a date, lot number, serial number, or other method, such as the designation "upon depletion of stock."

f) If applicable, the disposition of all raw materials, components, work in progress, finished goods, and distributed devices is assigned.

g) The responsibility for implementing the change is designated.

h) Any requirements for formal employee training/retraining are determined.

i) The document or document change is routed for review and approval. A signature matrix is often used to designate the individuals who are required to approve specific types of documents or changes to documents.

j) The document or document change is communicated to all affected parties.

k) The document is distributed to all persons responsible for operations affected by the document. Old documents are retrieved or removed from the system.

l) It is verified that the change has been implemented and that obsolete or superseded documents have been removed or steps have been taken to prevent their unintended use.

While not currently a routine practice in the medical device industry, the Quality System regulation requires manufacturers to ensure that those individuals or functions that originally approved a document review any changes made to that document. The use of a signature matrix, designating appropriate individuals and approvals, is one method of complying with this requirement.

CHAPTER 24. RECORDS (SUBPART M)

820.180 GENERAL REQUIREMENTS

The Requirement

820.180 General requirements. All records required by this part shall be maintained at the manufacturing establishment or other location that is reasonably accessible to responsible officials of the manufacturer and to employees of FDA designated to perform inspections. Such records, including those not stored at the inspected establishment, shall be made readily available for review and copying by FDA employee(s). Such records shall be legible and shall be stored to minimize deterioration and to prevent loss. Those records stored in automated data processing systems shall be backed up.

Discussion of the Requirement

Manufacturers are required to keep all records mandated by, or kept in order to comply with, the Quality System regulation, whether or not the record is product-specific. Whether maintained at the manufacturing site or at an off-site location, these records must be accessible to employees of the manufacturer and readily available for review and copying by FDA investigators. The FDA interprets "readily available" as available during the course of an inspection. A foreign manufacturer who maintains records at a remote site is expected to produce any requested records within 2 working days. In addition, records must be legible and must be stored so as to minimize deterioration and prevent loss.

When records are electronic in nature, backups are required to ensure retention, ease of retrieval, security, and accuracy. As with all automated processes, validation is required. Although a final policy for electronic signatures has not been released, FDA has indicated that when a signature or initial is a GMP requirement, the signature or initial may be handwritten or electronic. The use of stamps to indicate approval, which is a common practice in certain countries outside the United States, is also permitted. These issues are discussed in FDA's advanced notice of proposed rule making on the use of electronic signatures, which was published in the July 21, 1992, *Federal Register* (57 FR 32185), and in the proposed regulation published in the August 31, 1994, *Federal Register* (59 FR 45160). Therefore, FDA has not revised the regulation to use the term "identification," but the use of electronic signatures and stamps must be controlled and must take into account the concerns expressed in the draft electronic signature policy.

Industry Practice

While written copies of records are commonly used in the workplace, many manufacturers have converted to paperless systems in which records are generated, stored, and controlled electronically. These documents are made available to employees via personal computers at workstations or offices.

Most typical is for a manufacturer to centralize the document control function and to maintain a combination system of both paper and electronic records. Computers are used for the generation and storage of records, but paper copies are considered "official." It is still a common industry practice to circulate written procedures for review and signature by designated individuals.

While it is the responsibility of the manufacturer to decide what information to make available to FDA during an inspection, most manufacturers recognize FDA's right to review and copy records required under the Quality System regulation and provide investigators with broad access to procedures and records. Some manufacturers have inspection policies that address the policies, procedures, and records required under the GMP requirements and that specify which documents are and are not available during an inspection.

A typical issue involving records being readily available to FDA is how quickly a record must be retrieved, especially with respect to foreign manufacturing sites and records stored off-site. With the increasing use of computer networks and the Internet, retrieval of electronic records is becoming less of an issue. Even for those manufacturers without networks, records can readily be faxed from one location to another within one to two days. Off-site storage continues to be a problem, because many manufacturers have older records stored on paper and, as volume increases, must move them to remote locations. The issue of ease of retrieval is typically addressed in a manufacturer's records-retention policy.

The requirement to maintain legible records and to store records in a manner that minimizes deterioration and prevents loss addresses potential problems that both FDA and manufacturers have faced. Some examples of illegible records include records filled out in pencil or nonwaterproof pen and records filled out by hand by employees with poor handwriting. Loss of records may result from earthquakes and fires, and manufacturers are expected to have reasonable controls in place to prevent such losses, particularly when problems may be regularly anticipated. For example, storage in fireproof cabinets may not be expected routinely in most locations, but controls to ensure integrity of records and protection from earthquake would be expected of some California manufacturers.

820.180(a) CONFIDENTIALITY

The Requirement

820.180(a) Confidentiality. Records deemed confidential by the manufacturer may be marked to aid FDA in determining whether information may be disclosed under the public information regulation in part 20 of this chapter.

Discussion of the Requirement

The requirements of 21 CFR 20.20 provide for the fullest possible disclosure of FDA records, except for trade-secret and confidential commercial or financial information. Sections 20.60, 20.61, and

20.63 define the types of information that may be held confidential. Under section 20.27, the marking of records submitted to FDA as confidential raises no obligation by FDA to regard the records as confidential or to withhold those records from public disclosure. In situations in which confidentiality is uncertain and there is a request for public disclosure, FDA, under section 20.45, must consult with the person who submitted or divulged the information or who would be affected by disclosure before determining whether or not such data or information will be publicly disclosed. Judicial review is available, under 21 CFR 20.46, to any person whose request to hold information confidential is denied.

Industry Practice

Some manufacturers have inspection policies addressing how to determine whether or not certain types of company information are confidential with respect to disclosure by FDA. Manufacturers commonly mark as confidential any records subject to FDA inspection that contain trade-secret or proprietary information. Many manufacturers tend to be overly broad in claiming confidentiality, routinely stamping all procedures, drawings, and blueprints as confidential. A few manufacturers review documentation on a regular basis and carefully mark the information they believe to be confidential. However, the majority of companies address this matter only at the time a submission is made or documents are handed over to FDA.

Among the types of information that manufacturers want to protect are device specifications and proprietary manufacturing processes that would enable a competitor to produce a similar device. Information that FDA does not regard as confidential includes customer complaints (except the name of any patient or user), written procedures for compliance with GMP requirements, and DHRs (except to the extent that they contain proprietary process information or specifications).

The FDA makes every effort to protect information recognized by FDA as confidential and considers manufacturers' claims of confidentiality quite carefully. The FDA is required by law to release any information that does not meet the definition of information exempt from disclosure.

820.180(b) RECORD RETENTION PERIOD

820.180(b) Record retention period. All records required by this part shall be retained for a period of time equivalent to the design and expected life of the device, but in no case less than 2 years from the date of release for commercial distribution by the manufacturer.

Discussion of the Requirement

All records, including quality records, are subject to the requirement of this section. Records must be retained for a period equivalent to the design and expected life of the device, but in no case less than two years, whether or not the record specifically pertains to a particular device. Manufacturers are permitted to request a variance from the two-year requirement for devices with very short shelf lives, such as radioimmunoassay products. For a device with a long expected life, it is the responsibility of the manufacturer to determine the appropriate time period for record retention based upon the expected life of the device.

Industry Practice

It is implied in the regulation that a manufacturer will determine the expected life of a device in order to determine the required record-retention period. Assigning an expected life to a device is viewed by many manufacturers as a potential liability. Consequently, in actuality, required retention times are often chosen arbitrarily, allowing a grace period long enough to ensure that the specified time period will not be questioned when evaluated against the device produced. Regardless of how record-retention time is determined, the likelihood of field actions or other remedial activities is often considered, as is information on the device's fitness for use (e.g., complaints and service records).

Most manufacturers have a documented procedure for record retention, which includes a mechanism for disposing of records after the stated period has elapsed. Few manufacturers actually review records periodically and discard those records that fall outside the specified retention period. Consequently, many manufacturers keep records too long, and the majority of the records kept do not add value to their quality systems.

An important consideration for electronic record-keeping systems is maintenance of copies of obsolete or revised procedures. Many companies have a paper archive of procedures, which is, of course, an acceptable substitute for an electronic archive.

820.180(c) EXCEPTIONS

The Requirement

820.180(c) Exceptions. This section does not apply to the reports required by [section] 820.20(c) Management review, [section] 820.22 Quality audits, and supplier audit reports used to meet the requirements of [section] 820.50(a) Evaluation of suppliers, contractors, and consultants, but does apply to procedures established under these provisions. Upon request of a designated employee of FDA, an employee in management with executive responsibility shall certify in writing that the management reviews and quality audits required under this part, and supplier audits where applicable, have been performed and documented, the dates on which they were performed, and that any required corrective action has been undertaken.

Discussion of the Requirement

To ensure that manufacturers critically examine their systems and implement needed corrective actions and improvements, section 820.180 does not apply to reports of management reviews, internal audits, or supplier audits, which need not be provided to FDA during a routine inspection. However, these records may be available to FDA in litigation under applicable procedural rules or by inspection warrant when access is authorized by statute. Manufacturers are required to have written procedures for these activities, which must be available for routine review and copying by FDA.

The agency has the right to require a representative of executive management to certify in writing that the procedures required under sections 820.20, 820.22, and 820.50 have been followed, that the audits and management reviews have been performed, and that any necessary corrective actions have been undertaken.

Industry Practice

Most device manufacturers have written audit procedures that meet the requirements of section 820.22. These procedures are typically provided to FDA investigators upon request and without question. Although most manufacturers do not provide copies of audit reports to FDA, some routinely do.

Manufacturers certified by ISO already have written procedures in place for management review and supplier evaluation. Similarly to audit procedures, these procedures are provided to FDA investigators upon request. The majority of companies will not produce the results of management reviews or supplier audits.

The FDA has other means of assessing the adequacy of auditing and management review practices, such as the review of complaint files, incoming material and in-process acceptance records, and finished-device testing records.

820.181 DEVICE MASTER RECORD

The Requirement

820.181 Device master record. Each manufacturer shall maintain device master records (DMR's). Each manufacturer shall ensure that each DMR is prepared and approved in accordance with [section] 820.40. The DMR for each type of device shall include, or refer to the location of, the following information:

(a) Device specifications including appropriate drawings, composition, formulation, component specifications, and software specifications;

(b) Production process specifications including the appropriate equipment specifications, production methods, production procedures, and production environment specifications;

(c) Quality assurance procedures and specifications including acceptance criteria and the quality assurance equipment to be used;

(d) Packaging and labeling specifications, including methods and processes used; and

(e) Installation, maintenance, and servicing procedures and methods.

Discussion of the Requirement

Section 820.3(j) of the regulation defines "device master record," or DMR, as "a compilation of records containing the procedures and specifications for a finished device." The DMR, which is specific for the current design, must contain the necessary information for employees to perform both general and specific tasks related to the manufacture, testing, and release of a device, device type, or family of related devices.

The purpose of the DMR is to document the performance and configuration characteristics established for the device, components, packaging, labeling, quality assurance program, production, installation, maintenance, and service so that these activities can be controlled. The DMR must contain all the documentation necessary to meet this objective. The manufacturer of the device must have ready access to the DMR for each device manufactured.

The Quality System regulation does not specify how the information in a DMR must be organized or stored, although, as required under section 820.180, the information must be accessible to employees who use the records in their day-to-day job functions. Manufacturers are required to maintain a DMR for each device, device type, or family of devices. Any method may be used, provided that it facilitates reasonable access to the required documentation, control and identification of the documentation, and control of documentation changes.

It is a GMP requirement that the DMR be prepared, dated, and approved by a qualified individual to ensure consistency and continuity within the DMR. All documents contained in the DMR must be change-controlled, and any changes must meet the applicable requirements of section 820.40.

Device specifications required for the DMR include specifications for the finished device and for all raw materials, components (including labeling and packaging), and in-process materials, as well as the procedures for evaluating materials to ensure their adequacy and the forms on which inspection and test results can be recorded. These specifications may take the form of drawings or written specifications. Software specifications also must be included in the DMR.

Production process specifications include environmental specifications for air and water quality, when appropriate; specifications for all equipment; procedures for equipment qualification, operation, calibration, and maintenance; and record forms.

Production methods and procedures encompass all SOPs, assembly drawings, batch record forms, sterilization methods and procedures, and all other documents and procedures used in every stage of manufacturing, from procurement of materials through packaging and final release.

Quality control documentation consists of the procedures for inspection, evaluation or testing, and release of raw materials, in-process devices, and finished devices, as well as the specifications at each stage of evaluation. For any equipment used in inspection and testing, there must be written specifications, operation, calibration, and maintenance procedures, and forms for recording results.

Packaging and labeling specifications for finished device packaging, if different from incoming speci-fications, must be part of the DMR, along with procedures for receiving inspection, production, application, inspection, and release. Forms for the approval, production, and use of labels are required.

In addition, the DMR must contain the procedures and methods for installation, maintenance, and servicing of devices after they are released for distribution. This documentation must include the instructions provided both to the manufacturer's representatives and to users who install, maintain, or service the device themselves.

Industry Practice

Theoretically, if the DMR is constructed correctly, the contents could be taken to another location and used to produce a device which would be identical to the one produced at the original facility. A manufacturer may develop the DMR as

a) files or volumes containing the actual required documents and records;
b) a list or index of the documents and records that identifies their location; or,
c) any combination of these two configurations.

The GMP requirement that all documentation contained or referenced in the DMR be evaluated and approved by designated, responsible individuals before changes are implemented is typically met by having all such documentation under some type of formal change control. The actual ap-proval forms or documentation used to obtain approval are then included or referenced in the DMR.

To simplify DMR maintenance, most manufacturers maintain a change-controlled list or index that refers to or references all required DMR records. While it is not necessary to list every record in the DMR index, there should be traceability to each related document. Depending on the manufacturer, the DMR index may be in the form of an outline or a flow chart of the manufacturing process. Indented bills of materials are also commonly used as an index to the records making up the DMR.

Before the requirements of section 820.186, "Quality system record," were promulgated, manufac-turers typically created a "common" DMR index that included general quality system documents applicable to all devices or device families (e.g., audit procedures, change-control procedures, cali-bration programs, warehouse control methods, environmental specifications, cleaning procedures). The number of this index was then referenced in each specific DMR index, making it unnecessary to repeat all of the "general" document numbers.

The index may or may not designate document revision levels. Many manufacturers that use in-dices assign a document number and revision level to the index. The DMR index changes only when a new record is added or one is removed; the records listed in the index can change separately (new revisions) without the index being changed. However, if revision levels are not specified in the

DMR index, the manufacturer should have a system to demonstrate control over current revision levels. When a manufacturer uses a DMR index that specifies revision levels, such a system is not required because the entire index is updated each time a single document is changed.

Examples of records found in a DMR include

a) product and component specifications or formulations, including engineering drawings;
b) packaging and labeling specifications;
c) software specifications;
d) production.process procedures, methods, and specifications, including routine reprocessing;
e) sterilization parameters and procedures;
f) installation, maintenance, and service procedures;
g) test and inspection procedures;
h) environmental specifications and controls;
i) equipment specifications;
j) validation protocols and results;
k) bills of materials;
l) data sheets;
m) process flow diagrams;
n) operator's manuals; and,
o) service manuals.

For many manufacturers, the requirement that installation, maintenance, and servicing procedures be included in the DMR necessitates the generation of documents to guide their field forces. These activities, particularly maintenance and service, previously were simply handled on a case-by-case basis by qualified engineers.

Most companies that manufacture software devices or software-controlled devices already have procedures for software development, testing, and validation, because this information is requested in the 510(k) or PMA process. Accordingly, it should be a simple matter for these manufacturers to add the required information to the DMR.

820.184 DEVICE HISTORY RECORD

The Requirement

820.184 Device history record. Each manufacturer shall maintain device history records (DHR's). Each manufacturer shall establish and maintain procedures to ensure that DHR's for each batch, lot, or unit are maintained to demonstrate that the device is manufactured in accordance with the DMR and the requirements of this part. The DHR shall include, or refer to the location of, the following information:

(a) The dates of manufacture;

(b) The quantity manufactured;

(c) The quantity released for distribution;

(d) The acceptance records which demonstrate the device is manufactured in accordance with the DMR;

(e) The primary identification label and labeling used for each production unit; and

(f) Any device identification(s) and control number(s) used.

Discussion of the Requirement

Section 820.3(i) defines "device history record" as "a compilation of records containing the production history of a finished device." "Lot or batch," according to section 820.3(m), "means one or more components or finished devices that consist of a single type, model, class, size, composition, and software version that are manufactured under essentially the same conditions and that are intended to have uniform characteristics and quality within specified limits." Taken together, a DHR is a collection of records for a unit, batch, or lot of devices that includes information on the successful, or unsuccessful, completion of manufacturing steps and the results of receiving, in-process, and final acceptance activities, through distribution and, where appropriate, installation.

The DHR is intended to provide objective evidence that the requirements of the DMR were met and to provide information to facilitate failure investigations and corrective/preventive actions by providing traceability when the manufacturer is required to ensure traceability or when, for other purposes, the manufacturer requires identification of specific units or batches.

Each manufacturer is required to establish and implement written procedures to ensure that DHRs are maintained. All companies are required to produce a complete DHR containing certain minimum information, including dates of manufacture, quantities manufactured and released for distribution, and any identification or control number used.

The requirement that all labeling be included in the DHR reflects FDA's interest in increased control over labeling because of the many recalls that have occurred due to labeling errors. Requiring the DHR to include the primary identification label and labeling used for each production unit, as well as the control number or other identification used for each production unit, should, in addition to the labeling process controls required in section 820.120, help ensure that proper labeling is used.

Industry Practice

Virtually all manufacturers maintain a DHR, with the contents varying according to the segment of the industry, the size of the company, and the complexity of the device. The format of a specific DHR should be interpreted by the manufacturer, taking into account the complexity of the device and its manufacturing process and the raw materials, components, and operations that are most important to the proper functioning of the finished device. In the orthopedic device industry, for example, the major portion of the DHR often consists of a traveler card that specifies the major steps in the manufacturing process (e.g. cutting, grinding, polishing, cleaning), with each step being signed off or initialed by the operator. In the *in vitro* diagnostics industry, reagent DHRs often contain step-by-step instructions for measuring and mixing reagents, along with documentation of adjustments and test results, all of which are signed off by the operator. For sterile devices, the DHR contains information on the parameters of the sterilization process.

Most manufacturers conduct a review of the DHR to verify that it contains or references the data and information necessary to show that the required activities specified by the DMR were completed. This review, often coupled with product release activities, is intended to ensure that the product meets its quality attributes and that the records are in order.

In addition to ensuring that the DMR was followed during the manufacturing process, the DHR serves several other useful purposes for manufacturers. It contains information on incoming material acceptance, the manufacturing process, and testing results that can be used to perform trend analyses. Tracking or trending of quality data on materials and processes may identify production or supplier problems that require corrective action as well as areas of improvement for cost savings. The DHR also serves as the basis for investigating complaints and taking corrective action, because it provides a record of any shifts, changes, or variances in the manufacturing process that may result in problems with finished devices. Consequently, most companies maintain more than the minimum information specified for inclusion in the DHR.

In the past, many manufacturers did not keep representative samples of specific labels or labeling used. As a result of this GMP requirement, they are doing so in increasing numbers.

When device identification such as serial, lot, or control numbers is required (e.g., for critical devices, devices subject to tracking, *in vitro* diagnostics), this information is commonly recorded in the DHR. However, in many segments of the device industry (e.g., manufacturers of crutches, hospital beds, orthopedic hand instruments), serial, lot, or control numbers are not used. Manufacturers often make decisions regarding device identification based upon the need for traceability to identify problems or recall products.

Many manufacturers already have written procedures in place for the preparation and maintenance of both DMRs and DHRs. Typically, a DHR procedure specifies the content and format of the record and the review and approval process. Record maintenance and storage also may be addressed.

820.186 QUALITY SYSTEM RECORD

The Requirement

820.186 Quality system record. Each manufacturer shall maintain a quality system record (QSR). The QSR shall include, or refer to the location of, procedures and the documentation of activities required by this part that are not specific to a particular type of device(s), including, but not limited to, the records required by [section] 820.20. Each manufacturer shall ensure that the QSR is prepared and approved in accordance with [section] 820.40.

Discussion of the Requirement

The requirements of this section reflect FDA's efforts to harmonize the GMP requirements more closely with the international quality standards and to outline a hierarchy of the documents required for meeting the Quality System regulation. The intent is to allow the separation of the general quality system records from the device-specific records that make up the DMR. This approach allows the development of a quality manual, or similar file, that contains or references the more general documentation used for the overall planning and administration of activities used to define and implement the quality system.

Principles and requirements incorporated in this section of the Quality System regulation include

    a) quality planning;
    b) documented responsibilities and authorities;
    c) quality system procedures and instructions that are not part of a specific DMR; and,
    d) a quality system documentation outline or manual, as appropriate for a given manufacturer.

Industry Practice

Those manufacturers whose quality systems meet the requirements of an ISO 9000 standard typically have a quality system that includes most of the records specified in section 820.186. Manufacturers that do not have systems in place that meet the intent of the ISO standards also may comply already with many of the quality system record requirements. For example, procedures and documentation for device-specific quality have been required by the GMPs since they were first promulgated. Typically, manufacturers also have a documentation system in effect that ensures appropriate control over device-specific documentation. Many manufacturers have the same type of system and controls for general procedures as well.

The requirements of 820.20(b) indicate the appropriateness of a comprehensive set of documentation establishing quality responsibilities and relationships. A manufacturer can meet these requirements by providing organization charts and job descriptions if these documents relate the functions of each individual or group within a company to quality activities.

While not a specific requirement of the Quality System regulation, the development of a quality manual that includes the quality policy, a description of the organization, and a summary of the quality system procedures, with appropriate cross-references to more detailed documentation, can be utilized to meet the requirements of this section. The quality manual can be one document supported by several tiers of documents, with each tier becoming progressively more detailed; together, these documents define the quality system.

APPENDIX A: BIBLIOGRAPHY

APPENDIX A: BIBLIOGRAPHY

GENERAL

AMERICAN SOCIETY FOR QUALITY CONTROL:

Quality systems -- Model for quality assurance in design, development, production, installation and servicing. ANSI/ASQC Q9001-1994.

CEN:

Quality systems -- Model for quality assurance in design/development, production, installation, and servicing. CEN EN-29001:1987.

Quality systems -- Medical devices -- Particular requirements for the application of EN-29001. CEN EN-46001:1993.

EUROPEAN COUNCIL. *Medical device directives.* EC Directive 93/42/EEC. June 14, 1993.

FOOD AND DRUG ADMINISTRATION:

Compliance program guidance manual. Transmittal 95-30. May 4, 1995.

Inspection of medical device manufacturers. Compliance Program 7382.830, FDA Compliance Program Guidance Manual. May 4, 1995.

Medical device quality system manual: A small entity compliance guide. HHS Pub. No. (FDA) 96-4179.

Medical device GMP guidance for FDA investigators. HHS Pub. No. 84-4191. April 1994.

Medical devices: Working draft of the current good manufacturing practice (CGMP) final rule; Notice of availability; Request for comments; Public meeting. 60 FR 37856. July 24, 1995.

INTERNATIONAL ORGANIZATION FOR STANDARDIZATION:

Quality systems -- Model for quality assurance in design/development, production, installation and servicing. ISO 9001:1994.

Quality systems -- Medical devices -- Supplementary requirements to ISO-9001. ISO/CD 13485: 1995.

QUALITY MANAGEMENT

AMERICAN SOCIETY FOR QUALITY CONTROL:

Quality management and quality assurance standards -- Guidelines for selection and use. ANSI/ASQC Q9000-1-1994.

Quality management and quality system elements -- Guidelines. ANSI/ASQC Q9004-1-1994.

AMERICAN SOCIETY FOR QUALITY CONTROL *(continued)*:

Guidelines for auditing quality systems -- Auditing. ANSI/ASQC Q10011-1-1994.

Guidelines for auditing quality systems -- Management of audit programs. ANSI/ASQC Q10011-3-1994.

INTERNATIONAL ORGANIZATION FOR STANDARDIZATION:

Quality management and quality system elements -- Guidelines. ISO 9004-1.

Guidelines for quality plans. ISO 9004-5.

Guidelines for auditing quality systems. ISO 10011-1:1994, 10011-2:1994, 10011-3:1994.

Guidelines for developing quality manuals. ISO 10013.

DESIGN

DEPARTMENT OF DEFENSE:

Military standard system safety program requirements. MIL-STD-882C. January 19, 1993.

Procedures for performing a failure mode, effects and criticality analysis. MIL-STD-1629A. November 1980.

Technical reviews and audits for system equipment and computer software. MIL-STD-1521B. June 4, 1985.

FOOD AND DRUG ADMINISTRATION:

Deciding when to submit a 510(k) for a change to an existing device. Draft 2. August 1, 1995.

Design control guidance for medical device manufacturers. Draft. CDRH, March 1, 1996.

Device recalls: a study of quality problems. HHS Publication FD 90-4235. CDRH, January 1990.

Do it by design: An introduction to human factors in medical devices. Draft. CDRH, March 1, 1996.

ODE Guidance for the content of premarket submissions for medical devices containing software. Draft. Office of Device Evaluation, CDRH, August 12, 1996.

Preproduction quality assurance planning: Recommendations for medical device manufacturers. Office of Compliance and Surveillance, CDRH, September 1989.

Reviewer guidance for computer controlled medical devices undergoing 510(k) review. Office of Device Evaluation, CDRH, August 1991.

INSTITUTE FOR ELECTRICAL AND ELECTRONICS ENGINEERS:

Guideline to software design descriptions. IEEC 1016.1-1993. March 1993.

Recommended practice for software design descriptions. IEEE 1016-1987. March 1987.

Recommended practice for software requirements specifications. IEEE 830-1993. December 1993.

Software engineering standards collection. 1994.

Standard for developing software life cycle processes. IEEE 1074-1991. January 29, 1992.

Standard for software project management plans. IEEE 1058.1-1987.

Standard for software test documentation. IEEE 829-1983. December 1982.

Standard for software verification and validation plans. IEEE 1012-1986. September 1986.

INTERNATIONAL ELECTROTECHNICAL COMMISSION:

Analysis techniques for system reliability -- Procedure for failure modes and effects analysis (FMEA). Publication 812. 1985.

Fault tree analysis (FTA). Standard 1025. 1990.

Medical electrical equipment, Part 1: General requirements for safety. IEC 601-1. Second Edition. 1988.

INTERNATIONAL ORGANIZATION FOR STANDARDIZATION:

Quality management and quality assurance standards -- Part 3: Guidelines for the application of ISO 9001 to the development, supply, and maintenance of software. ISO 9000-3:1992.

ACCEPTANCE ACTIVITIES

AMERICAN SOCIETY FOR QUALITY CONTROL. *Sampling procedures and tables for inspection by attributes.* ANSI/ASQC Z1.4--1993.

AMERICAN SOCIETY FOR TESTING AND MATERIALS. *Practice for choice of sample size to estimate a measure of quality for a lot or process.* ASTM E122-1989.

BHOTE, KR. *Supply management, how to make U.S. suppliers competitive.* New York: AMA Membership Publications, 1987.

DEPARTMENT OF DEFENSE:

Sampling procedures and tables for inspection by attributes. MIL-STD-105E.

Sampling procedures and tables for inspection by variable for percent defective. MIL-STD-414.

TAYLOR, WA. *Guide to acceptance sampling.* Lake Villa (Ill.): Taylor Enterprises, Inc.

PRODUCTION AND PROCESS CONTROL

AMERICAN NATIONAL STANDARDS INSTITUTE:

Standard for protection of electrostatic discharge susceptible items: Personnel grounding wrist straps. ANSI EOS/ESD Standard No. 1, August 1987.

Standard for protection of electrostatic discharge susceptible items: Grounding -- Recommended practice. ANSI EOS/ESD S6.1--1991.

AMERICAN SOCIETY FOR QUALITY CONTROL. *Calibration systems.* ANSI/ASQC M1-1987.

ASSOCIATION FOR THE ADVANCEMENT OF MEDICAL INSTRUMENTATION:

Medical devices--Validation and routine control of ethylene oxide sterilization. 3rd ed. ANSI/AAMI/ISO 11135--1994.

Sterilization of health care products -- Requirements for validation and routine control -- Industrial moist heat sterilization. ANSI/AAMI/ISO 11134--1993.

Sterilization of health care products--Requirements for validation and routine control--Radiation Sterilization. ANSI/AAMI/ISO 11137--1994.

FEDERAL STANDARD. *Clean room and work station requirements, controlled environment.* FED-STD-209E.

FOOD AND DRUG ADMINISTRATION:

Application of medical device GMPs to computerized devices and manufacturing processes. Office of Compliance and Surveillance, Division of Compliance Programs, November 1990.

Contract sterilization. SMA Memo No. 16. DSMA, August 24, 1982.

Guideline for the manufacturer of in vitro diagnostic products. Division of Compliance Programs, Office of Compliance and Surveillance, CDRH, February 1990.

Guideline on general principles of process validation. CDRH and Center for Drugs and Biologics, May 1987.

Guideline on sterile drug products produced by aseptic processing. Center for Drugs and Biologics and Office of Regulatory Affairs, June 1987.

In vitro diagnostic products inspectional guidelines. Division of Compliance Programs, Office of Compliance, CDRH, and Division of Clinical Laboratory Devices, Office of Device Evaluation, January 24, 1986.

Preproduction quality assurance planning: Recommendations for medical device manufacturers. Office of Compliance and Surveillance, CDRH, September 1989.

Sterilization of medical devices. Compliance Program 7382.830A, FDA Compliance Program Guidance Manual. May 4, 1995.

INSTITUTE FOR ELECTRICAL AND ELECTRONICS ENGINEERS:

Guideline to software design descriptions. IEEC 1016.1-1993. March 1993.

Recommended practice for software design descriptions. IEEE 1016-1987. March 1987.

Recommended practice for software requirements specifications. IEEE 830-1993. December 1993.

Software engineering standards collection. 1994.

Standard for developing software life cycle processes. IEEE 1074-1991. January 29, 1992.

Standard for software project management plans. IEEE 1058.1-1987.

Standard for software test documentation. IEEE 829-1983.

Standard for software verification and validation plans. IEEE 1012-1986.

INTERNATIONAL ORGANIZATION FOR STANDARDIZATION:

Accuracy (trueness and precision) of measurement methods and results -- Part 1: General principles and definitions. ISO 5725-1:1994.

Accuracy (trueness and precision) of measurement methods and results -- Part 3: Intermediate measures of the precision of a standard measurement method. ISO 5725-3:1994.

Aseptic processing of health care products. ISO/TC 198 171.

Quality management and quality assurance standards -- Part 3: Guideline for application of ISO 9001 to the development, supply and maintenance of software. ISO 9000-3:1991.

MORRIS, AS. *Measurement and calibration for quality assurance.* Prentice Hall.

NATIONAL AERONAUTICS AND SCIENCE ADMINISTRATION. *NASA standard for clean room and work stations for microbially controlled environments.* NASA Publication NHB 5340.2. 1967.

PRODUCT CONTROL

INTERNATIONAL ORGANIZATION FOR STANDARDIZATION. *Packaging for terminally sterilized medical devices.* ISO/DIS 11607.

MONITORING AND FEEDBACK

FOOD AND DRUG ADMINISTRATION. *Medical device user facility and manufacturer reporting.* 60 FR 63578-63607. December 11, 1995.